MORE THAN
EYES CAN SEE

Published in Great Britain and the United States in 2007 by
MARION BOYARS PUBLISHERS LTD
24 Lacy Road London SW15 1NL

www.marionboyars.co.uk

Distributed in Australia by Tower Books Pty Ltd,
Unit 2, 17 Rodborough Road, Frenchs Forest, NSW 2086, Australia

Printed in 2007
10 9 8 7 6 5 4 3 2 1

A CIP catalogue record for this book is available from the British Library.
A CIP catalog record for this book is available from the Library of Congress.

ISBN 978-0-7145-3142-7

Set in Bembo 11/14pt
Printed in Wales by Creative Print and Design

MORE THAN EYES CAN SEE

A nine-month journey through the AIDS pandemic

by

Rhidian Brook

MARION BOYARS
LONDON • NEW YORK

For Gabriel and Agnes,
who made it possible to see much more.

'Write my name somewhere.'
Pascal Kyengo

Contents

Prologue

'Only connect' – E. M. Forster

This book has unusual provenance. It was someone else's idea and only one part of a much bigger idea at that. It came my way via a long, serendipitous chain of human connections set in motion by a woman who lived ten thousand miles away...

In the Autumn 2003, Nikki Capp, a Melbourne mother of two, member of the Salvation Army and part-time employee of drug company GlaxoSmithKline was troubled by a big subject and a needling question: HIV/AIDS and what are you going to do about it? As a corporate affairs manager for GSK (who made the antiretroviral drugs (ARVs) taken by HIV/AIDS patients) and through her own awareness of the Salvation Army's HIV/AIDS work, she was often stepping into the penumbra of the pandemic's shadow. She was part of two monolithic – almost antithetical – organisations, linked by the common ground of HIV/AIDS.

One night, she had what she called a 'waking dream' in which she saw five people sitting around a table: herself; the General of the Salvation Army; JP Garnier (the then global head of GSK); her husband Nick (who worked for a micro-financing organisation); and Rupert Murdoch, the head of News Corporation. The people around the table were having a conversation about HIV/AIDS.

By her own reckoning Nikki was 'a nobody' in both GSK and the Salvation Army but she interpreted this dream as a commission to get to the tops of these organisations, orchestrate a meeting between them and pitch the idea of them working together to address the global HIV/AIDS issue. For the next two years, she set out to persuade these VIPs to take seats at the table of her dreams. She already had one vital connection to an Australian doctor called Ian Campbell, the head of the Salvation Army's International Health Services and something of a seminal figure in HIV/AIDS response work; and there were openings, through her own and her husband's work, to GSK and the world of micro-finance. But the journey was not a straightforward stroll through a line of open doors; there was much scepticism, some scoffing and a number of nearly-but-not-quite encounters that required doggedness, a 'truck load of faith', and 'constantly telling myself that I wasn't crazy'. After two years it was just about possible to imagine reserving at least three of the seats at the envisioned table. The elephant not in the room was Murdoch.

Nikki's mentor at that time was the retired former head of the Salvation Army, General Eva Burrows – a legend in Salvation Army circles – and a woman who, in her role as world leader of the Army, had made powerful friends. One such friend was Dame Elisabeth Murdoch, the mother of Rupert Murdoch.

Despite her age (ninety), Dame Elisabeth was sharp on events and a great champion of the 'Salvos' (as the Salvation Army were known in Australia); she was happy to meet Nikki to talk about such an important issue. Nikki travelled to Dame Elisabeth's house outside Melbourne and after a drive around the grounds in the dame's buggy, she began to explain what she thought she was trying to bring about. She felt, as she often did telling people about her dream, 'like a total idiot,' but Dame Elisabeth saw meaning in the peculiarity. She took Nikki's materials – detailing the nature of the Salvation Army's worldwide HIV/AIDS response – and a letter requesting a meeting with her son. She wrote 'Rupert's' home address on an envelope and handed it to Eva so that she could write to him personally. 'When he sees my handwriting, he'll open the letter.'

Months passed and Nikki was again wondering if her idea was a dream too far when, in January 2004, she received a message through Eva Burrows that Murdoch was willing to meet her. That April, the media mogul gave 'the woman from Melbourne who had had a dream' as much time as he usually allotted to world leaders. As she stepped over the threshold of the News Corp building, Nikki recalled the line she'd read from the Book of Esther and that she'd written in her diary months ago as an encouragement: '…who can say but you have been elevated to the palace for just such a time as this?'

The king of News Corp was gracious and practical; he expressed genuine concern for the HIV/AIDS situation and he was struck by the nature of the Salvation Army's response to the pandemic. He indicated his willingness to bring News Corp to the table to discuss how the four proposed partners might do something together. He said he would nominate someone in his organisation to help Nikki explore ways of developing a partnership. A meeting was actioned for the Autumn in London.

In November 2004, Nikki and Dr Ian Campbell met with James McManus, the head of TSL education, Nigel Hawkins the Health Editor of *The Times* – who had a particular expertise in HIV/AIDS – and Simon Willis, a managing director at the TSL group.

Nikki and Ian had talked about what they wanted to say beforehand. 'In our heads it sounded good: statistics about HIV/AIDS and poverty didn't drive action; but stories and real life experience did. By helping people experience that, maybe in some way we might move them to act. We wanted them to help us help "the man in the street" realise that people living in poverty have the same aspirations, dreams, resilience and innate capacities to survive and to prosper, as does anyone living in a wealthy country and that understanding this was a key part of our response to HIV/AIDS.'

But what sounded worthy and good in their heads sounded confused and imprecise when pitched. Salvationists use a lot of jargon and have a predilection for acronyms (they are an army after all). If the substance of the work was deep the describing of it was flat. As Ian Campbell began to talk about local 'facilitators' and 'motivators', Community Counselling, Income Generating Activities (IGAs) and Psycho Social Support (PSS) activities, the eyes of the corporate-speak-savvy executives began to glaze over. After hearing them out, James McManus raised a finger: half Salvation Army salute (pointing to heaven); half 'Please stop!'

'This is great – the work sounds wonderful and we want to help – but I haven't the foggiest idea what you're talking about.'

Ian and Nikki's hearts sank. All this treasure but no easy way of sharing it.

'That's our problem,' Nikki said. 'We need someone to help us put the deeds into words.'

It was then that Simon Willis suggested the idea of writing a book. It wasn't the full realisation of the dream, but Nikki felt that perhaps it was a part of it. They began to discuss how, who, when and where. 'Immersion in different communities around the world in different continents,' 'drawing up alongside the infected and the affected.' Dr Campbell and Nikki knew some good people in the field who might be able to 'facilitate the collecting of stories'.

James McManus put up an interventionist finger again.

'There is no way you or anyone in your organisation can write this book. You have to find someone else to write it; to "facilitate the collecting the stories", as you put it. "Do you know anyone who might want to do that?"'

…Just when you think you're in the middle of your own story - playing the main role, speaking your familiar lines, going through your habitual motions – you find yourself part of someone else's story; a story that has been going on for some time and in which you have a small role to play.

Author's Note

This is an account of a journey I made with my wife Nicola and our two children, Gabriel and Agnes, between January and September 2006, to the heart of places affected by the HIV/AIDS pandemic.

The task has fallen to me to write about what I saw and I can't entirely – nor would I dare – speak for my family. But because we were together 24 hours a day, seven days a weeks for nine months, there were moments when we became an eight-eyed, eight-legged creature, seeing and experiencing things as one. For this reason I occasionally switch from the singular 'I' and 'me' to the collective 'we' and 'us'.

It was unusual to send a whole family on a journey like this. The fact it happened this way is, in part, down to the inspiration and insight of the Salvation Army AIDS response team who knew already how much deeper we might go if we went as a whole family; but it was also due to my family's intrepid and naturally curious personalities; and their willingness to take a risk. And I am hugely glad they came with me. Apart from not being able to cope with the loneliness, I am not sure I would have got access to situations and acceptance from people to the degree that we did had I been a writer travelling solo.

I have recorded the journey in the order we made it rather than trying to keep to a strict geographical taxonomy. Largely for reasons of climate and convenience, we decided upon a route that started in Africa, in the community of Kithituni,

Kenya; then, to avoid the sapping heat we went to India – to Mumbai, Satara, Mizoram and Calcutta – in February; and back to Kenya, on to Rwanda and Uganda, before heading south to Zambia, Zimbabwe and South Africa. We then crossed the ocean and several latitudes to Hong Kong and Mainland China before finishing the working part of the journey in the United States, in Los Angeles.

The common thread in this seemingly random selection of cities and countries was that they were all places severely affected by HIV/AIDS where the Salvation Army had a presence. The confluence of these two things determined our choice of destination and provided the *raison d'être* for this venture and this book. Before I was about to embark on writing this book I found myself envying those authors who decide upon a focused geography – like Siberia, Patagonia or Route 66 – and then write about it. Our route was on the map but its unifying, thematic characteristic was not topographical, lingual, political or economic; it was epidemiological, and the cause and effects of this particular disease weren't always easy to see. HIV/AIDS lead us to places, subjects and themes we hadn't necessarily planned on visiting (and worthy of whole books in their own right); so, if occasionally I step off the designated road, I hope that the reader won't be thrown or disappointed. In picking up and following the blood red thread of this disease we often found it entwined with other threads that made up a larger, complex tapestry in which many issues overlapped and bled into each other.

Commissioner Hezekial Anzeze – the executive leader of the Kenyan Salvation Army – told us to expect this. He said: 'You are on a hunt for a particular animal. While you are on this trail, you will come across the trails of other animals and want to follow them, too. And so you should, because they are part of the hunt. The difficult thing is that the animal you are after is elusive and difficult to find because it is hidden most of the time; you will sometimes feel that this animal does not exist because it can't always be seen. But it is there. You just have to look with more than your eyes.'

Rhidian Brook
London, May 2007

The Road Was Red

At first, the road was red and our shadows were short. Our feet were our transport and conversation our sustenance. The road we were walking sometimes wound out of sight for a while before rising again into view and cutting through the distant hills. The people used the road to meet with bosses and brothers, get to water pumps and *rendez-vous* with lovers. The road was vein and artery, carrying the freight of human endeavour to and from the cities, towns, villages and communities. It was an innocent conduit for the transport of material goods and simple kindnesses, as well as a benign passage for the deadly disease we were tracking. Sometimes the road changed from red dust to jet macadam and the transport from foot to bike to bus to sleek sedan; but it made no difference: the best of routes only served to carry the worst of cargo more quickly.

Eventually we had to come off the road because it wasn't the road we needed to follow; it was the people on the road, going back to their huts and *shambas*, church meetings, community conversations, bars and brothels. For these were the places where HIV/AIDS had its formation. This pandemic had not spread via some sinister plot or random mosquito bite; but through the most basic and intimate kind of human transaction. Just as this pandemic had its roots in relationships so it was possible to find its antidote wherever one or two were gathered.

In January 2005, I took the first wavering steps on this road as I walked to the International Headquarters of the Salvation Army in Blackfriars to a meeting to discuss whether I would be willing to write a book documenting the Army's response to the HIV/ AIDS pandemic. I had actually decided that I would not be taking up the potential commission. I was going along out of deference to my wife Nicola (who thought we should do it) and politeness to the Salvation Army and my friend Simon Willis (who had suggested my name to them in the first place). As I walked across the Millennium Bridge towards the International Headquarters of the strange, idiosyncratic organisation I knew little about beyond the clichés of brass bands and comforting cuppas, I paced out my mini mantra for not going:

Career, ignorance, family, health.

In that order.

Any one of these objections provided a sound enough reason not to go; their aggregate seemed conclusive. I thought I was clear on this but as I got closer to the scripture-embossed, glass-fronted building, I felt my resolve swaying like the aluminium construction beneath me. By the time I was close enough to read the words of the one I claimed to follow, written in lazered-glass across the entrance – 'I am the light of the world. Whoever follows me will have the light of life' – my mind was a fog of indecision.

I had been reading a book called *In Darkest England and the Way Out*, written in the main by the founder of the Salvation Army, William Booth. Published in 1891, it is a summation of Booth's beliefs and observations about what was wrong with the world (England) and what he hoped to do about it. It had an energy, anger and authority which was breathtaking; but what set this book apart from other rants about what is wrong with the world was its lived criticism, its practicality and its prescience: it didn't just dwell on the malady, it offered a remedy – a set of remedies in fact, many of which were scoffed at at the time but have since become a reality: a citizens advice bureau; women's enfranchisement; shelter and food for the homeless; work for the out of work; and some that are just coming into being: the travelling hospital; a poor man's bank; co-operative, organic farms. This was the work of a man who was not a philosopher or social engineer theorising from behind his desk about the iniquities of life whilst offering no way out; it was the thinking of a man who had clearly engaged with the worst that the world and mankind had to offer and who believed there was something that could be done about it. The title of the book – *In Darkest England and the Way Out* – was an arresting counterpoint to the then hugely popular *In Darkest Africa*, Henry Morton Stanley's account of his (ultimately murderous) exploration of that continent. England was then febrile for tales of adventurers cutting a swathe through the thick jungle of unchartered lands, tales that mixed excitement and wonder with dread and horror, all wrapped up in a safe sense of superiority. Booth's point was that you don't have to go that far – to Africa – to find the dread and horror when it was right here on your doorstep.

Were he here now, Booth might be amazed to see how much his country had dragged 'the submerged tenth', as he called it, from the gutter; grateful too, to learn that the citizens of this country enjoyed some of the benefits that he once proposed. But he'd have been appalled by the new statistics that were shaming our civilisation. That 'submerged tenth' of England had been replaced by a submerged two-thirds out in the world, beyond these sorted shores in the countries that we had once claimed to 'discover'. If some of the old, world-wrecking diseases had gone away they had been replaced by new afflictions, like HIV/AIDS, that were killing people on an even greater scale and, as always, it was the poor who were taking the full force of it.

Booth was particularly exacting with the Church of his day; keen to separate out the respect-obsessed, cultural Christians from true followers; he hated the former's lukewarm commitment, their smugness and disregard for those being crushed by the world. In his book he wrote: 'in the struggle of life the weakest will go to the wall, and there are so many weak. The fittest, in tooth and claw, will survive – all that we can do is to soften the lot of the unfit and make their suffering less horrible than it is at present. Is it not time that they (the Church) should concentrate all their energies on a united effort to break this terrible perpetuity of perdition and to rescue some at least of those for whom they profess to believe their founder came to die?'

I was a supposed believer, like Booth, in a redemptive plan; someone who really does see the Church, at its best, as central to that plan; and that it's the poor and the lost who we are called to serve; but I was walling myself behind the accepted, sensible reasons for not going on a journey like this and greying my argument with another excuse masquerading as modesty: 'the world is full of enough do-gooders; what difference can you make anyway?'

If I was looking for omens to reinforce my stance, I was in the wrong bit of town. Just outside the headquarters, a man was selling copies of *The Big Issue*. When the editor of that magazine – John Bird – was asked what advice or wisdom he could pass on to people wanting to do something about the state of the world he said: 'Keep asking the naïve questions: "Why are there so many poor people in the world? What are you doing about it?"'

I sidestepped the man selling the magazine and walked into the International Headquarters of Booth's Army building for my meeting. Minutes later I was seated around a table with six people involved with the Salvation Army's response to HIV/AIDS including their International Health Consultant, Dr Ian Campbell, his wife Alison and Sue Lucas, a consultant to UN/AIDS. Dr Campbell, started to outline the nature of the job and what would be required.

'We'd like someone to see for themselves what it's like; someone ready to live within these communities long enough to feel the loss, the grief, the breakdown of social structures and get close enough to hear and see what people are doing to overcome the problem; someone able to find the stories of hope in the midst of seemingly overwhelming despair. It won't be easy or always comfortable, they'll see things they won't believe and won't want to believe. But the best way – the only true way – for this person to be a witness is for them to be there.'

I ventured my ignorance, suggesting that there were surely people more expert than me who could take on the job.

'The world of HIV/AIDS has enough experts,' he said. 'We don't want a statistician or a specialist, we just want someone to go and see it and find the stories. Go expecting to learn and you will find the story.'

'What is the story?'

'This thing has its formation through relationships – people searching for belonging or significance; and it's through relationships that people can find a solution to this pandemic. But to see this you have to be there. Get your hands dirty. Smell it. Live it. You will have to immerse yourself for a considerable time.'

(His neutral 'someone' had become the assumptive 'you'.)

'How long will it take?'

'Nine months to a year.'

'What about my family, my wife and two children?'

'Take them with you. Where you're going being a family will be an asset.'

I shook my head. Not to say no, but at the sorry sight of my sensible reasons not-to-go evaporating into the ether.

The doctor then looked at me, fixed me with his blue eyes, and asked:

'Can you think of a good reason why you wouldn't do it?'

Going Where It's Darkest

A year later, I set off with my family on a nine-month journey that would take us to eleven countries in three continents – into the very heart of the AIDS pandemic.

The night before going we had looked at my son's atlas and circumnavigated the world with our fingers. Between the familiar world maps showing Temperature, Population and Religion, were the new maps charting recent human concerns: Environmental Issues, Travel and Tourism; there was also a map showing the percentage of adults living with HIV/AIDS. Where once I had looked at a world that was colonial pink, my children were now staring at a world shading from lilac to deep violet, indicating the spread and depth of a pandemic. But for a pure white Australia and Scandinavia the whole world was under a purple shadow.

I traced our intended route with my finger, starting in lavender Britain, scratching a course south to amethyst Kenya. Across to mauve India; then back to the artichoke heart of Africa – Rwanda and Uganda – before plummeting south into the puce of Zambia, Zimbabwe and South Africa. Two ocean spanning finger strides took us to the controlled lilac of China and the USA, before my nail traced a line full circle back to England and home.

'We're mainly going where it's darkest,' Gabriel said.

For the next nine months 'the deep purple places' were going to be our home.

We started where it started, in Africa and in the Sub-Saharan band of countries that lie on the equator, where the first great wave of AIDS appeared and crashed over twenty years ago. Our first base was to be in a Kenyan community on a red road just like the one in the picture on the cover of the book I had just read before leaving and had with me in my rucksack.

That book, called *The Ukimwe Road*, was by the Irish travel writer, Dervla Murphy, a woman once described as 'the toughest female traveller of her age'. The road Ms Murphy took had led her from Kenya to Zimbabwe, via Uganda, Tanzania, Malawi and Zambia. She made the journey, by bicycle, in the early 1990s, intending to get away from personal difficulties and hoping to 'enjoy a carefree ramble through some of the least hot areas in Sub-Saharan Africa'. But the further she pedalled the clearer it became that the purpose and subject matter of her journey and book were not going to be what she thought; everywhere she went she encountered talk of a mysterious threat of *Ukimwe* (a Swahili word for AIDS) and the devastating effect it was having on the people. By the time she reached journey's end in Zimbabwe she had found her theme.

When I was eighteen, at a time when AIDS was seen as a disease restricted to affecting the gay community in San Francisco and had not even been given its final, contentiously agreed acronym,* I worked in Stanfords, a map and travel bookshop in Covent Garden. One day I was asked to assist a middle-aged lady who was looking for maps to Madagascar with a view to cycling around that massive African island in the Indian Ocean. The woman was the famous travel writer Dervla Murphy.

Twenty-four years later, my godfather – Jeff Barker – sent me the same book. He had just been to Ghana to work for

---

* The travel-writer, Bruce Chatwin, who died from an AIDS related illness in 1989 wrote: 'the word AIDS is one of the cruellest and silliest neologisms of our time. Aid means succour, help, comfort yet with a hissing sibilant attached to the end it becomes a nightmare.'

VSO* reviewing the various AIDS NGOs (Non-governmental Organisations) there and he thought the book would be helpful. But when I received it and saw the cover depicting a painting of a red road bisecting yellow grass, spotted with acacia trees – the trees that say 'Africa' – I remembered that I had seen this book before and that I had, in fact, been given it by my wife, Nicola. I searched our bookshelves and found it. Inside, Nicola had written a date – '11th March, 2002' (my 38th birthday) – and a suggestion: 'For another possible (Brook–Sulman) adventure!'

At that time, we knew nothing about this coming journey. My wife had given me the book because she knew I'd once met the writer and also because it was time for us, as keen travellers, to go to the continent we had always been too busy, too afraid or too lazy to visit. Four years later, the prophesied adventure was under way and, like Murphy's, it turned out to be a journey unlike the one we might have anticipated; a journey that would take us to Sub-Saharan Africa and way beyond. By the time we set our feet down on a real red dust road, HIV/AIDS was no longer a mysterious rumour whispered in villages or contained to a community in an American metropolis, it had become a full blown ululation of pain and grief that was echoing right around the planet.

On the night flight, we were abuzz with anticipation and medicine. Our anti-malarials were coursing through our blood and our biceps still ached from our final round of jabs. We were setting off on our journey, inoculated against a host of deadly diseases into the realms of a disease for which there was no cure. We had had four months of knowing for sure we were going and the idea of it had become almost too big to carry. We had read on and around the subjects of HIV/AIDS – and Africa. We had learned about prevalence rates and transmission; we had explained to

---

* VSO or Voluntary Services Overseas is an international development charity that works through volunteers.

Gabriel and Agnes – and reminded ourselves – how HIV passed from one person to another; we'd familiarised ourselves with the political arguments over interventionist approaches versus non-interventionist. And we had tried to get a sense of what life would be like in the communities we were going to. But reading medical texts, Chinua Achebe or Laurens van der Post only primed one part of us. Like soldiers trained for war through simulated combat, we were prepared for anything but we knew nothing.

When I was ten, I was given a beautifully illustrated copy of *The Swiss Family Robinson*. I still had the book and had read it to the children before we set off on this journey. It is, of course, an idealised, bucolic story and this was a different kind of adventure; but we were not unlike the Robinsons: green, middle-class, 'civilised', privileged, going into a world for which we were ill-equipped and unprepared, not knowing what we were going to find there – or what we were going to discover about ourselves.

We were met, in Nairobi, by April Foster, a member of the Salvation Army's Regional Facilitation Team. April is an American who has worked in Africa for sixteen years and who, for the last twelve years, had lived in Kenya. Also there to greet and escort us to our new home was Mark Mutungwa, a young man who hailed from Kithituni, the rural town where April was building a house in which we were going to live. At the time of our arrival, this house was still being constructed. April had not yet lived in it herself, but she felt it was a good place for us to start: comfortable and safe enough for a green family to stay; raw and in the sticks enough to get close to the daily rhythms and disruptions of life in a rural African community and to see, close-up, the effects of the disease and the people's response to it.

It was unusual – radical really – for someone who had never met us to offer us a house they themselves had not yet lived in, but it was a foretaste of the simple generosity of spirit we were going to encounter in that place. It was also – we were going to discover – a gesture in keeping with the nature of a woman who held 'things' lightly and had other ideas about how you spent your time and your money. April did not fit into any category I recognised. She was certainly no colonial looking to exploit the country's resource for her own gain. For a white, single, foreign woman to build a house in a rural community with little infrastructure, poor water access and little power there had to be some other motivation.

April's house – our new home – lay some 150 miles south-east of Nairobi. Once we got beyond the billboards for mobile phone companies and 'Trust' condoms and the outlying hotels and the first truck weigh station along the Mombasa Highway, the landscape opened out and the great Acacia plains of the Masai land spread out like a sea with a horizon as infinite as any ocean's. Driving away from the capital we had the sensation of going out to sea, our vessel getting smaller and our voyage feeling bigger than we had supplies for.

In the 1980s, the British government had backed a big campaign informing the public of the dangers of having unprotected sex. AIDS was depicted as an iceberg, a largely hidden hazard, the full weight and ballast of which lay beneath the surface, ready to sink every happy ship that came its way. It was a frightening campaign and presumably effective in getting the sexually promiscuous British to wear condoms because the disease never reached the rates of infection and prevalence that the admen threatened. AIDS and icebergs make for an incongruous simile in equatorial Africa, but as we drove across the hot plain, I imagined the pandemic lying just out of view, below the surface, waiting to sink the next passing ship.

Mark drove steadily, mindful of the poor road surface and the high risk driving style of the *matatus** and trucks that run

---

* A *matatu* is so called because a *tatu* (meaning three) used to be what it cost in shillings to get a fare.

the gauntlet of East Africa's main trade route. The road – in a terrible state considering its significance to the nation – carried the freight, imports and exports of many countries; it was both artery and vein, conveying goods back and forth from heart to hinterland. The men who drove the trucks that carry the goods were not unlike sailors crossing a dangerous sea, away from home for long stints and susceptible to all the risks and temptations of loneliness and lust. All kinds of cargo is transported along this route, including the deadly freight of the HIV virus that through those drivers found an easy transit across the continent and into the outlying towns and villages.

Some say that the low life expectancy in African countries accounts for the careless driving. This is impossible to prove, but of all the possible ways we might die on this journey a car wreck was the most likely. We had only been in Kenya four days and had read of three major road crashes with a collective death toll of one hundred. I kept my eyes fixed on the potholes and measured the overtaking spaces between the oncoming trucks, whilst talking to Mark about the state of the nation.

President Kibaki has his hands full: a big scandal involving corrupt ministers driving expensive fleets of four-by-four vehicles, a drought which was killing people in the north of the country, and the ever-present battle against the unseen killer of HIV/AIDS. Mark spoke of these things in gentle, unaccusing tones but he was passionate about them. He was a strikingly beautiful man, inside and out. He had the high cheekbones of the Swahili-side tribes and an easy, languid grace and humility that you don't encounter much in our own pumped-up, self-promoting culture. At first I thought I might be romanticising this, seeing things through the green eyes of the newly-arrived, but we soon discovered that these qualities were not uncommon. In fact, meeting people of grace and humility was to become such a regular feature of our journey that we came to expect it and were shocked when we didn't find it.

We had heard from Ian Campbell that Mark was a key link in the chain of little connections that had led to the Salvation Army's AIDS response in Kithituni. Without him April would not have decided to build a house there and we would quite likely not be making this journey.

I asked him to tell us how he'd got to this point in his life.

Seven years ago, HIV/AIDS was devastating his community and people were asking what could be done. The Salvation Army district officer at the time was a woman called Rebecca Nzuki. Rebecca had just come from the Kibera – the Nairobi slum – where she had been working among a group of women involved in commercial sex-work. She'd encouraged these women to meet and support each other financially and as they shared their experiences, a common thread emerged: most of them were HIV positive but had no means of support. Rebecca saw that they as a group of people would have to be their own support network. The women started to pool resources, visit each other, get medicines when they could. Without knowing it these women were modelling a communal method of response that was to provide a template for future HIV/AIDS response in Kithituni and beyond. In Kithituni, Rebecca transferred everything she had learned in the Kibera and began visiting the infected and the affected in their homes. This got people talking and then participating and she soon had 'a team' of local volunteers assisting her. Mark was one of the first to volunteer. He began to encourage others – his family, his friends and neighbours – to participate in the 'home visits' and 'income-generating projects' and 'community counselling' sessions. Getting his family involved was key. Mark was one of thirteen children. His mother and father – Agnes and Jonathan – were a totemic couple in this district. Jonathan was the head of the clan but also a quartermaster in the Salvation Army and the longest serving member of the Kithituni corps; he had been a Salvationist for fifty years. He was a man of influence – nearly all of it benevolent. It was Jonathan who had given April the plot of land on which to build her house – itself an unusual step, and the day Jonathan changed his mind about whether it was acceptable to openly discuss HIV/AIDS and sex in and around church was a key moment for the community in galvanising them to face up to and get to the root of what was killing them.

The response in Kithituni was infectious and it spread quickly through the region to a point where fifty communities had some level of community-led HIV/AIDS work. Hearing the good rumours emanating from this district, the regional team came to see the work and discovered that what was happening in this typical African community had something to teach a wider world.

Mark suddenly stopped talking and pointed to the sparse copses on the roadside: there, towering over the bushes like upside down trees, stood three giraffes. He pulled the vehicle off the side of the road and we all got out to get a closer look. We cheered at the sight of these animals – so other-worldly, so unlikely – that we had only ever seen in zoos. Mark said that it was unusual to see them so close to the road; the lack of rain was driving animals out of their usual habitat in search of water and vegetation but he had never seen them so far north.

'Will we see a leopard here?' Gabriel asked.

People come from all over the world to see the wildlife here and Kenya, with its long grass plains and acacia trees and wildlife, provides the archetypal mental landscape that forms many people's idea of what Africa is. Looking at these beasts and seeing how our children reacted to the sight of them, I did feel a thrill of recognition; something in me was saying now you're really here. But the feeling was checked by a kind of sadness. Our own safari – a Swahili word that means journey – was not going to involve much conventional sightseeing. We had not come to admire the beauty of the wildlife or even the landscape; we'd come to live in places tourists avoided, and to spend time with people who usually get overlooked by visitors too busy chasing the aesthetic to really notice, let alone connect with them; we had come to look for an animal more elusive, less pretty and far more deadly than any leopard.

At the road town of Sultan Hamud, Mark turned the vehicle left and onto an 'A road' of pure red dust. Our house was only six miles along this road but this stretch took half an hour to cover. For Mark terrible roads were a fact of life and he seemed impassive at the halting progress we made. We didn't mind because it was part of the new; part of the adventure. Months later, putting a man called Pascal into a packed *matatu* in order to deliver him to the nearest hospital forty miles away, the state of these roads would seem less like a thing to love. For now though, they were the finest, most elemental roads – the red dust road of archetypal imagining.

We turned off this tributary onto a slightly narrower, even more dust-laden road. Little houses made from bricks and straw punctuated the view, while the people – mainly women and children – stood in front of their homes waving, selling, looking, smiling. More people were gathering at this intersection to collect water from the main waterhole. About twenty people with jerry cans and plastic tub barrels waited their turn to fill up with water that was there because an Italian company had built a pipeline from Mount Kilimanjaro some seventy miles to the south-east of us. When our bottled water from the Nairobi supermarket ran out this is where our own drinking water would come from.

This last stretch of road to our house was imprinted with deep truck tracks that were compacted enough for people to ride their bikes in. The rest of the road was deteriorating fast. Mark said this was caused by the trucks from Nairobi coming to take sand from the dried-up riverbed back to the city for concrete. Our house – April's house – was just off this road, about a mile along it. The house was unlike all the other houses we had passed on the road here but it was not incongruous. Its character – its rondaval shape – was African even if its scale was Western. We were going to be living in relative luxury: the house had a generator that gave us power for three hours a day; we had a pit latrine that was more than fifty yards away from the accommodation; and we had running water. We were about forty minutes walk – twenty minutes bike ride – from the main town, the Salvation Army church, the market; and our nearest neighbours, just over the way, were Mark's parents – Jonathan and Agnes – and his brother and sister-in-law Jacob and Margaret and their two sons Martin and Richard. We couldn't have been in a better neighbourhood.

The house was still not finished and part of the welcoming contingent was made up from the building team who would be billeted on the land until their work was done. The Mutungwa family were also there to greet us: Jonathan a sprightly, impish seventy-year-old, still vigorous and nattily dressed in slack linen suit and trilby and Agnes, (handily having the same name as my daughter) quite regal and with a look of such strong, piercing love it made you want to confess your sins there and then, repent and change. Agnes had born thirteen children and her body shape showed this; but her face was quite sublime, all chiselled intelligence and a smile and teeth that dazzled. She spoke no English and our Kiswahili was fledgling but there was much understanding between us, communicated through hands clasped and cheeks kissed and a laugh that came from some deep place of knowing.

Words of greeting were exchanged and translated by Mark and Margaret. Then a tray of biscuits, sodas and water was brought out and put on the table. I helped pass drinks around (I was host and guest now) but when I handed Agnes a glass of water she took it, raised it and paused. I wasn't sure why she was pausing and thought perhaps I had broken some arcane protocol, or that I should have offered her a soda or the bottled water that we had

33

brought with us from Nairobi to drink instead of this water that came from the big plastic bin in our kitchen. But then I saw that her eyes were closed and that she was praying. She prayed for this glass of water for much longer than I have seen anyone pray a grace, even graces prayed before feasts and weddings. It was a holy toast to the God who had brought us here safely and who had made it possible for this water to fall from clouds into rivers and through pipes into wells to be poured into buckets and carried on bicycles to this place.

'Where Are All the Sick People?'

'Much unseen is also here' – Walt Whitman

In those first few days and weeks, we were a bit like those poet-naturalist-farmer-writers, taken aback by the beauty of the red earth roads, the mountains in the distance, the hills in the foreground, the birds, the just-right heat and the wood-smoke and sweat smell that you think you recognise even though you've never been here before. My first message home was not – as I had anticipated – a bulletin of woe, it was more an ecstatic yell. I remember asking the question if we had ever really been alive until this moment; and feeling annoyed that for such well-travelled people we had not come to this continent sooner.

When people told us that Africa gets into your blood I had the sense they meant the landscape. It is – when you see, touch and smell it – a revelation: it makes you realise that the rich plasma you've had coursing through your system is a thin, anaemic watery substance and that to survive here on the iron-zinc red earth and beneath the instant heat of the just risen sun, you're going to need a transfusion.

But if the landscape got our blood up; it was the people that got under our skins.

Despite our uncertainty about fitting in, it turned out that we had credentials: we had come to a town where every other woman seemed to be called Agnes; this bought us instant cachet; we were white and from England; that made us exotic

35

and (still) respected. We were living in April's house; that made us esteemed friends; being with the Salvation Army made us brothers and sisters. But the thing that made our acceptance in the community instant and unreserved was that we were a family. Ian Campbell had predicted that being family would 'accelerate our integration' in the community; it would 'enhance the engagement'. And so it proved: Jonathan and Big Agnes would swing by on their way to market to check we were okay; Margaret and Jacob's son, Martin, would come to play with Gabriel and Agnes (football at first and then Game Boy). Gabriel when not being home-schooled by Mum would go to school with Martin. Hoards of children would pitch up and hang out – some of them all day. George the Baptist would stop off for tea and a chat. Lelu would fix up our water and show us how to kill the army of ants that walked in through the front door at exactly seven every night; the Major lent us a bicycle. On the 45-minute-walk to market, we would shake the hands of a hundred people and practice the local greetings. 'We don't say *Jambo* – that's what tourists say. We can say *Mambo*. Reply: *Poa*. (Cool). Or *Habiri Yacko*. Reply: *Mzuri sana*. Or *Sasa*? Reply: *Fitte*. That's Swinglish. Or *Kamba*: *Wacha!* (only to someone younger than you). Reply: *Aaahh!*' By the time we had said 'hello' and 'fine thank you' for a week, bought two goats at Friday market (we called them Malarone and Larium after the malaria tablets) and been to church, the freedom of Kithituni had been granted.

The normality was deceptive. I recognise now, cooled down and distanced, that some of this enthusiastic initiation was the shock of the new and relief at escaping the vile English winter; but it was more than that. Our non-travel to Africa to date had been, in part, a matter of protective postponement. Our world had given us sensible reasons not to visit the apparently diseased and mayhem-riddled continent; and it had planted deep roots of fear in us. When we arrived we were so prepared – visually at least – for the worst that it was a shock not to see dead people lining the route. When you have been weaned on the milk of disaster to a point where you cannot conceive of Africa, or its people, to be anything other than face down in that red dirt, it's actually a surprise to see people upright and going about their day, smiling and joking, smartly dressed, clean.

After a week of being there, Gabriel asked me: 'Dad, where are all the sick people?'

At first, AIDS did not seem to us to be the obvious problem. The people had more conspicuous 'life and death' issues to deal with and in the first days, even weeks, it was these issues that fought for our attention and sympathy: the drought, the resultant lack of crops, the terrible roads, the difficulties of not having free secondary education, malaria, the lack of access to water.

We talked about water a lot.

When we arrived, it hadn't rained properly in this area for two years. In the north of the country there was famine and I had seen on the news that there was a big relief operation going on near the Sudanese border. Up there it is nearly desert, but here the land was meant to be more fertile and, with the short rainy season approaching, the people were getting twitchy about what another year without the rain would do to them. The pipeline from Mount Kilimanjaro provided water for the whole region but it was not sufficient to irrigate the *shambas* (fields or plots where food is grown) and all around us the crops were drying out and withering.

There was plenty of water, beneath the land, but to get to it you needed to use equipment beyond the means of a community like this. 'Why don't the government build bore holes?' we asked. For the cost of a Mercedes four-by-four vehicle favoured by the ministers in the Kenyan government you could drill ten bore holes in this district alone.

'The government have promised to do this, but we don't know when it will happen.'

When we weren't talking about water, we talked of education.

That first week a man knocked on the open door of our house and stood waiting on the porch. He was nervous and most likely embarrassed – passing his hat through his hands like a steering wheel in the gesture of someone who was going to ask for something – but his need, whatever it was, was greater than his pride and he was clearly swallowing a lot of that by coming to see the *muzungu** family who by now most people in the community knew were living in April Foster's house and, being from London, would certainly have more than enough money to help with the occasional individual request.

We did not want to make him feel any more uncomfortable than he already was. My wife offered him a chair and a glass of water and a biscuit that he accepted with the humble reverence that Agnes had shown. Then, in broken English, he explained to us the nature of his problem, a problem that we would hear repeated throughout the journey: he did not have enough money to pay for his daughter to complete her secondary education and would appreciate 'any assistance we could give'. (I have with me now a small collection of correspondence from people including a letter from a man in Uganda asking if I might help pay for his sons to attend university.) In Kenya, primary school education had only been free since President Kibaki had come to power and the United Nations had loaned Kenya the money to pay for it; secondary education however was not free which meant either that many children between the ages of eleven and eighteen simply didn't go to school or families, already struggling financially, having to make inordinate sacrifices to send perhaps one of their children to a secondary school. The sums asked for were not small – even for us – but we said we would talk about it and see what we could do. The man thanked us. He didn't feel

---

* *Muzungu* – white.

good about asking us and he appreciated our time. He worked hard but he had three children to raise and since his wife had died things had been very difficult.

'How did your wife die?' I asked him.

'She died. From AIDS.'

Even a dry riverbed leads towards the same sea.

After a few days of playing with the children around the house, our own children began to tell us which of their new friends were orphans whose parents had died from HIV/AIDS.

It was just as Hezekial Anzeze had told us: just when you're on the trail of something else you'll come across the trail of the thing you're looking for. This image of AIDS as an elusive animal had seemed ungainly at the time, given the observable damage the disease had wrought across the world. But this picture was to prove more and more apt, the further we travelled. This virus goes about its business quietly, sowing away in private places and then appearing, sometimes years later, to claim the payment. It's a particularly brutal bailiff and it fractures bodies, relations and communities; but although it has highly visible and visceral consequences its 'acquisition' happens behind closed doors, in intimate settings; and its destructive activity remains invisible for a time, unseen by those outside and unknown even to the person who is infected. Poverty, poor roads, lack of rain, poor education, bad politics, inadequate medical facilities, were all helpful allies but to really spread successfully, the pandemic required, relied really, on totally invisible, very human elements – desire for intimacy, betrayal, loneliness, infidelity, corruption, despair, lust, abuse, cruelty, greed.

We had entered two big myths at the same time: AIDS and AFRICA, and in order to see what was really going on – to get to a place between the poetry and the catastrophe – we were going to have to dump a lot of baggage, the metaphor, the imagery, the literature – the whole weight of argument and opinion we had with us in our heads and rucksacks – and use our own eyes. Engaging with people and their stories was the only thing that would get us beyond the myth and metaphor to the thing itself.

'Aspire To Inspire Before You Expire'

'You and whose army?'

I didn't have to wait long.

On my first day of working with the Kithituni local response team I went to the funeral of a man who had died of AIDS. They were going to go and show their support for the dead man's family – a wife and five children – as well as the extended community. Going to funerals was an important part of the team's work and this was their fifteenth AIDS related funeral in the last six months.

I met with the team* at ten in the morning at their 'office' – a corrugated tin-roofed, concrete hut next to the Salvation Army church. This day's team (it would vary according to availability, employment, weather, health) consisted of Georgie-Porgie, Johnnie Boy, Anton, Onesmus, (all young men in their early twenties) Margaret and Catherine, (both mothers and daughter-

---

* As well as the pioneering work done by Rebecca Nzuki, the idea for these teams came out of the Salvation Army's work under the aegis of Doctor Ian Campbell at the hospital in Chikankata, Zambia, where the first case of HIV/AIDS appeared in the 1980s (see later chapter – 'A Short History of Care'). Back then, the hospital had been used to treat leprosy and the policy was to isolate the sick. For two decades the hard work of facilitating family inclusion and destigmatisation had happened. When HIV/AIDS appeared, it was clear that hospital-based care was not the solution – people needed help at home with family and neighbours so the hospital decided to go out to the sick and conduct what were called home visits. This too, because of the numbers of the infected, became unsustainable, and so the hospital decided to equip and encourage the community to respond to those who were sick themselves.

in-laws of Jonathan and Agnes); Oral Roberts (named after the great preacher) and me. Oral was not a Salvationist, he was an Anglican, but for many people life around here had got too short for these kind of denominational differences; like the effect war has on people of different class and political persuasion, AIDS was having a unifying affect.

Today the gathering was bolstered by the presence of an old woman called Mama Safi – who wore a Stars and Stripes bandana – and three other elderly ladies who between them had formed a co-operative garden market selling vegetables and fruit, as well as milk. They had just purchased a cow called Miriam and the milk was being given to the AIDS orphans in the community. The last to arrive was Joseph, also a young man in his early twenties, who had been to deliver okra from his *shamba* for Friday market. That completed the team.

We formed a circle – 'a beeg, beeg, circle' – with the white plastic chairs forming the outer ring. Johnnie Boy spoke a benediction and then started to clap and sing and the hot hut soon swelled with the sound of these voices giving thanks for what they had, which to my eyes wasn't very much. The first devotional they sung was the one that we sang most frequently and became the 'team anthem' out on the road. It had a beautiful melody that was easy to harmonise and the words – in Swahili – had a powerful refrain.

hakuna mungu kama wewe (x 3)
There is no god like you
nimetembea
I have travelled
nimetafuta
I have searched
nimezunguka
I have turned all round
hakuna na hatakuwepo
None and there shall never be another God like you

The thanking-of-God continued way beyond my own capacity for thanking Him but I was fast having to recalibrate my sense of what to be grateful for and with it my capacity for thankfulness. We were beginning to learn that here, each day got through was something to be celebrated and a person could find in the smallest provision – milk from the cow, a soda, a glass of water – something to be grateful for.

After the devotionals I was asked to formally introduce myself and say why I was here. It was no bad thing to be asked this question – easy to presume you know the answer. I said that I was here to try and understand the problem of HIV/AIDS and see how they as a community were responding to it. Thankfully no one seemed thrown by this.

Then Onesmus, who was the acknowledged team leader of the Salvation Army Kithituni response team, reminded everyone of the team's *raison d'être*: why they were here; what they were trying to achieve. He spoke clearly, in a leaderly way, although there was in this introduction and his phraseology a strange hybrid of the naturally eloquent African way of speaking and the consultancy aphorism the West exports to the world.

'The responsiveness of the community is what we are trying to inspire.'

'We believe that what we are doing is helping others to realise their human capacity and so inspire others.'

'By staying connected to community we are transferring our knowledge to help them realise their capacity to respond.'

His words were backed by the statements and words written on A2 flip-chart paper and that decorated the peeling walls of the hut. Marker-penned statements of intent: 'Aspire To Inspire Before You Expire'; 'Care Leads To Change.'

Half way into the meeting I could not stop myself from thinking: 'Is this it? A handful of people, a little faith, some by-rote management-speak slogans, and some songs? Is this an adequate response to the world's greatest health crisis?'

If, at first, I found myself inwardly mocking the language (its proximity to advertising) in time I'd hear it differently. The slogans and the pep talk were, of course, of more profound consequence than any equivalent discussion that may have occurred in a brainstorming meeting; and these people weren't discussing a sub-plot for a murder story or a headline for a life assurance company, they were trying to fight a war against a pandemic with whatever weapons they could – including words. Maybe where there is a lack of money, language (which costs nothing) has to take up some of the slack.

In her book *Aids and its Metaphors,* Susan Sontag takes exception to the use of the military metaphor when describing disease – particularly AIDS. She argues that the effect of military thinking about sickness and health over-mobilises, over-describes, and 'powerfully contributes to the excommunicating and stigmatising of the ill'. William Booth however had little doubt that he was engaged in a war – a war against poverty, vice and sin – which was why he started an army to fight it. In *In Darkest England*, he wrote in the preface: 'The progress of the Salvation Army in its work amongst the poor and lost of many lands has compelled me to face the problems which are more or less hopefully considered in the following pages. The grim necessities of a huge Campaign carried on for many years against the evils that lie at the root of all the miseries of modern life, attacked in a thousand and one forms by a thousand and one lieutenants…'

It was hard to think of the ragtag assembly of boys and girls and men and women gathered here in this hut in such martial terms. They were less an army – more a guerrilla force. Or perhaps a home guard. No one had press-ganged them into this war; they were all volunteers, doing it for nothing and for love.

Suddenly it started to rain and the drops smacked onto the tin roof like a thousand little drummers and we all stopped. When we realised that it was actually raining there was spontaneous thanksgiving in song. The rain was just a short, teasing shower but it brought hope, and that was a commodity as valuable as rain.

We were soon walking the red road: Johnnie Boy, Georgie-Porgie, Onesmus, Lelu, Joseph, Catherine, Margaret and me. (The old ladies went back to their homes as they had animals to husband.) The funeral we were going to was in the next village, about a two hour walk away, and we walked slowly because by now the sun was fully up and there was no cooling wind coming off from the hills. The road was wide enough for all eight of us to spread right out across its full span; occasionally we would break up to make way for a *matatu* minibus heading for the market in Kithituni or a truck going to the dried-up River Mikayu bed to harvest sand for a concrete company in Nairobi. It had not rained here properly for two years now and the dust lay thick like a brick-red snow. Up ahead a trailing brown cloud announced the approach of a vehicle coming our way and we split to the sides of the road to watch a *matatu* pass. These mini-buses were officially meant to carry fourteen, but once off the main highway drivers would pick up as many as could squeeze in. This one passed us with slide side door open and men hanging from the runners and the team waved to some people they knew; there must have been 25 packed in the vehicle. We then reformed the line and started to talk about the man who had died.

He was in his mid-thirties. He had five children. He died from AIDS. Although the man had died of AIDS – technically the thing that finally killed him was pneumonia. Strictly speaking, no one dies from AIDS itself for AIDS is not an illness but a medical condition whose consequences are a spectrum of illnesses. The fact that people with HIV/AIDS usually die from one of the opportunistic infections – TB, pneumonia, diarrhoea – means that the cause of death is not always clear because it is deliberately obfuscated out of shame. Even now, years into a pandemic which had killed over a million people in a country that was as aware of HIV/AIDS as any, a family would rather say their deceased relative died from pneumonia than from *Ukimwe*.

The team had been visiting the deceased for four months, counselling him, taking him food or medicine; but their work was not over. Their presence at the funeral was an act of solidarity but also a statement of intent. Their simply being there said – in a way that words couldn't – that 'we are here to honour the death of this person – yes, a person who has died of a disease that some still think brings shame.'

The team were known in the district as 'the AIDS guys' but the boys had given themselves an unofficial moniker: The Chi-ang Mai, after the famous mountain resort in Thailand where the prevalence of HIV/AIDS had been dramatically reduced thanks to a programme of community response initiated by colleagues and partners of the Salvation Army there. The name had a cool ring to it but I couldn't quite get away from the fact that they had named themselves after a place synonymous with Western, hedonistic, promiscuous sex-tourism. But I kept these thoughts to myself. We needed to get to know each other a bit better before talking about stuff like that.

It was just after midday when we arrived at the house of the dead man and there was already a crowd of about a hundred there, most of them sitting in the thin shade of the acacia trees and on the smooth, hard ground between the thorn bushes that bordered the man's straw hut. Before joining them we were duty bound to meet the local clansman – chief – and say who we were and where we were from. The chief was seated with three other men and wearing a white cotton shirt and wide brimmed straw hat. He looked weary; he had attended too many funerals lately; this disease was taking up too much of his thought and ruining the rhythms of the life he knew; but he seemed encouraged at our presence and wanted to know where we were all from. It turned out that the dead man's wife was Johnnie Boy's sister, which made the dead man Johnnie Boy's brother-in-law. Johnnie had not mentioned this either in the meeting, or on the road when we were chatting. It was as if it went without saying that when you go to a funeral of someone here you were going to be related to them in some way.

We then took our places on the ground, just in the shade of a tree where bicycles were stacked. These bicycles were like the bicycles we would have ridden in the 1950s – gearless, sturdy and black. They were either made in China or India. (It was hard to find anything that was made in Kenya.) They were decorated with bright coloured paint patterns, embroidered seat cushions and extravagant mud flaps, some with mottos or scripture on them. 'I'm The Boss.' 'The Lord Is My Shepherd.'

Women brought over trays of *ugali* and soup-stew. *Ugali* is cooked maize flour and it looks like blocks of porridge crossed with mashed potato and tastes like neither; it's a staple stomach filler though and thick enough to use as cutlery with which to eat the soup which was a thin stew with potato and chunks of gristly meat floating in it; but we gratefully ate and drank, talking in whispers and watching the people gather. The crowd were forming a semicircle around the dead man's straw and mud house. At the edge of the plot a mound of earth and dust indicated the spot where the man was going to be buried.

I could see, off to one side, a Catholic priest in sky blue cassock, sitting slumped and sad, looking at scripture, preparing himself for the service. Presumably the man who died had been a former member of his congregation. I was curious to see how the priest might negotiate the difficult task of honouring the dead, the family and sticking to the truth of what really happened here.

'Do these people know how this man died?' I asked Onesmus.

'Yes. But not everyone.'

'Will the priest say how he died, during this service?'

'Maybe. I hope so.'

He began the service with a prayer. Next to him some relatives of the man stood in a huddle but none of them were crying. Not so long ago, there would be more ceremony than this and grieving wails and ululations would fill the air; but these were exceptional times. This disease mocked mourners with its frequency and made tears a luxury; the proper rituals were truncated by expediency and the funerals had become emotionally mute.

There was no sound now but the voice of the priest and the wind in the washing. It was not a cool wind nor strong enough to shift the small clouds that hovered tantalisingly over the hills and which had earlier teased us with a shower. If only it were strong enough to move the clouds from the hills to this place and let loose some rain. But it was all dry here: too meteorologically dry for rivers and too emotionally dry for tears.

The priest looked weary, like a man whose tank of hope was close to empty from driving too far and too many times down this same road. But he appeared to steel himself, as if raising his own faith so he might once more be able to tell the people who had come here that death doesn't have the last word in this world.

He started by challenging the gathered to think about their own death. 'Have you made a will?' he asked us. 'Have you thought about your own end? Are you ready to face what is coming?' He didn't shout this question; he asked it, gently nudging us all. 'People do not want to speak about the end. When you ask if they have a plan they don't want to speak about it; but are you prepared?'

It was a good question to put to people still alive, their hearts pumping blood and permitting them to stand at the graveside of the dead; just in case they fall into feeling that what happened to this man was some kind of anomaly, an aberration that cannot and will not ever affect them; by asking this question the priest drew us closer to the dead man's plight and made it all our concern.

I had made a will before leaving home. It was the first will I had ever made and I made it because I thought it wise, given the amount of travel, the types of transport we'd be using and the kind of places we were going to; there was a chance of us dying on this journey. Unlike the man we were burying, I was insured to the hilt and in the event of my death (my insurance company tripled my premiums upon declaring the intended geography of our travels) I calculated a handsome pay out to my wife and children. 'Yes,' I thought, when the priest asked the question; 'I have made a will. I had thought about my death and I was prepared.' But I knew this wasn't the kind of preparation the preacher meant.

He continued to probe, using the occasion to good effect. This, in his mind, was the correct way to honour a man who had died from AIDS: let the people know what happened here so that they will not go the same way.

'How *did* death come to this man?' he asked. 'It wasn't a sudden thing. A random sickness. A bite from a mosquito. An accident. It came in the midst of his life. Maybe in a moment of great pleasure and satisfaction. Even through the good pleasures this life affords, death lurks, waiting for us. So when we bury this man, let us not just think about his death; let us think about our own death; for a wise man is ready for death and is not afraid.' There was no glossing over or covering up; no obituary spin, no silence as to the causes of the dead man's dying. The tone was: it could be you and I being lowered into this that pit. He then called on the community to come together and support the orphans – five of them – in the way that they used to 'during the times of our grandparents when we came together to support those who are weak.'

And then the coffin was lowered into the pit by six men and prayers were said. The old women sang a dirge while the men shovelled the earth from the mound back into the pit. The earth thudded insensitively on that coffin and the men disappeared from view as the dust from the shovelling enclosed them. Had anyone been passing they might have mistaken them for workers on a building site. There would be no discreet filling in of the sod later, once the mourners had gone; things had to be buried quickly in this land and everyone was now a sexton. It took six men half an hour to complete the task, with wheelbarrow and shovel and watching them I thought that there was no easy way to make this look dignified and maybe that's a good thing. Dust to dust on dust over dust.

On the way home, my companions discussed what would happen to the children left behind. They said that it was up to the community to support the widow and the children, a difficult task as the lack of rain and drying *shambas* meant that the community was already struggling to support itself; but there were no real alternatives. They discussed how they might contribute food – onions, tomatoes and okra – to the family from the *shamba* that they were going to cultivate – a *shamba* irrigated by water from the bore hole that April Foster had dug. I couldn't figure out how these people were able to think so optimistically. Here they were, on a hot Monday, in a rainless land, going to a funeral partly because they had no other work, walking past dried out crops, trying to think of ways to support children out of what little they had when all they had in their pockets was Hope.

Sex In Church

We followed the sound of the big drum and it drew us to the market place. There, in a 'beeg beeg' circle, some of the Salvation Army (Kithituni Corps) band were playing an 'open air meeting' 'drumming up' the people before the Sunday morning service. They wore uniforms of white with faded blue lapels and they stood out in the mud and dust of the brown market place. The women had the bonnets, the men the peaked caps. When the drumming stopped they sang accompanied only by a tambourine. Some passers-by watched and one or two old ladies joined in with the singing. Then a girl with close-cropped hair stepped out into the middle of the circle, accompanied by an old lady. The old lady was steering the girl to the centre of the circle because the girl was blind. The blind girl took her spot and then stared off away over our heads, her own head tilting as if to listen to see. Then she started to preach. She was about fifteen years old but she had an authority way beyond her years and I found myself shifting uneasily, as if she might single me out and challenge me: 'who are you and what are you doing here?' She was blind and yet she seemed to see us all and her words had twice the search and reach because of what she couldn't see.

Before we set out on this journey, the Salvation Army was no more than an affectionate joke to me. An Army of Fools. Brass bands in winter. Collection boxes. Soup kitchens. Uniforms. And it was strange to see the joke replicated in another land, albeit with its own cultural tweaks. The story of how this Victorian movement translated to the cultures of the world is worthy of another book. But if it is a joke it is a practical joke and its practitioners willing fools.

When the drumming up finished the band proceeded to the church itself. Already there was a large gathering of people, many in uniform, although not all pristine or regulation. A very old lady came to shake my hand. She was diminutive, like a scrawny child, and she was wearing 'her own' Salvation Army uniform, a hybrid of the formal white and the faded African and all the better for that. Her white lace shirt might have been worn by a Victorian child at a christening around the time when William Booth was founding this movement back in the late 19th century (a movement that eschewed such formalities as infant baptism and communion).

Mama Safi – the old lady with the bandana – was there. Mama Safi said she was 101 years old. She looked too sprightly to be senile then again she looked too sprightly to be one hundred so perhaps it was a selective amnesia, a prerogative of age. Mama Safi's earlobes drooped and holes the size of coins indicated a tribal, pre-Christian past. She took my hands and spat on them and then she pulled me to her and spat on my chest by way of blessing. I looked at her hands and they looked like the hands of a 101-year-old – you can see in them the lines of her life. Some say that it is the hands of old women that are damming the flow of man-made-destruction engulfing this world.

Inside the church some of the boys from the local response team were seated at the back of the congregation. We all waved to each other. But there was no hiding at the back for us. We were honoured guests and we took our places of honour in the front row where everyone could see us. Then the officers entered and we all stood and launched into the first chorus. After the chorus we sang a hymn, more Victorian English than Kenyan, and then went back to a chorus. We were then introduced to the congregation – the community – and we stood to say some words which were translated by Jonathan into Kamba and by the Major into Swahili. Then the Major's wife performed a kind of rallying-cry-call-to-arms-admonishment all in one.

'Some people have not been giving enough this month and that is not good,' she said.

The Salvation Army may not like ritual but they make one of their giving. The soldiers brought their tithes to the front desk, one by one. Those who had not tithed were outed by the Major. This transparency about who gives what made for good drama and the plot thickened when Jonathan stood up the front and started the pledging of food for the orphans. He said it was time for us to do something about the orphans and he set an example by pledging a sack of maize.

'Who will pledge?' he asked. 'Who will give something?'

Someone else said they would buy a crate of long life milk cartons; another said they would bring onions and tomatoes from their *shamba*. A list was made. I raised my hand and pledged a sack of beans. Others bid their gifts and promised to bring them to the service next week, but Jonathan wasn't satisfied with the demonstration of support so far; he wanted and expected more from the congregation.

And? And? He coaxed them with his expressive arms.

These people didn't have much. It seemed unreasonable to ask them to give more but he persisted and after a time more hands were raised and food promised. This process took up nearly forty minutes. It was the antithesis of the embarrassed offering I am used to seeing in church, where the wooden offering tray is hot-potatoed across the line and people furtively drop in their coins. Here the process of tithing is something alive and vital; it is not individual it is communal; it is a matter of life and death.

I felt good about myself as I placed our own offering in the tray at the front, an offering I deemed commensurate with our relative wealth, but also a generous amount because it surely constituted the largest single contribution in the tray and maybe even equalled the combined total of the entire congregation of two hundred. But then I saw the collection tray (an up-turned tambourine) being taken to the treasurers for accounting and in amongst the coins I noticed two just-laid white eggs sitting in it, the chicken's feathers and droppings mottling their shells, and I felt ashamed of myself.

The service went on too long and the corrugated tin roof cooked us all, but order and pattern are needed to keep chaos outside the door and despite my reservations about religion, I was beginning to see why the dressing up, the display, the order, are vital. This coming together was a half religious duty; half expression of hope and belief. The things said and the transactions made here – seen and unseen – had great bearing on the community. It was in this building that Jonathan publicly changed his mind about talking about sex in church.

No respecter of traditions or age, AIDS has had a hair-ruffling effect on the sensibilities of the churchgoer and the establishment. Were Africa not such a Christianised culture, this might not be an issue; but with 70% of the population attending a church congregation of some kind and the Church providing three quarters of the social services in the entire continent, the Church's response to AIDS was and still is of vital consequence. For better or worse, people here listen to preachers and priests.

At first, the religious interpretation of the disease was limited to the notion that this was some kind of plague sent by a God who was punishing people for their sexual transgressions; but this judgemental and spiritually bankrupt interpretation wasn't going to suffice for a response when people started losing brothers, fathers, mothers whose only error was to sleep with their husband, children whose only sin was to be born with the virus in their blood. The divinely punitive interpretation was also a get out – a lazy avoidance of blame and excuse for non-engagement with the real issue: 'I'll let God deal with them while I will get on with my righteous life.'

The sexual nature of the virus also placed a disastrous taboo on the subject. Even though it is a fact (a fact continually lost in the red noise of debate) that in 95% of cases the virus is acquired by two people doing something that is as natural as the equatorial sun rising and descending each day. If you were a virus that depended for your spread on ignorance, taboo, stigma, fear, condemnation and general obfuscation then how much would you love the Church to remain silent. 'The longer you don't acknowledge me and my ways,' the virus might say. 'The more people I will kill. Go ahead, don't talk about the real reason people acquire me; see how many I will destroy; don't talk to your children about sex because it's difficult and embarrassing and not what your fathers did – and then see how I will lay waste to a whole generation who were never told; keep thinking that somehow God can't handle you discussing sex (something He presumably intended) and that he will be embarrassed and offended by such talk, and watch your congregation dwindle through want of simple conversation.'

But people in and out of church were having the discussion. When the regional response team – including Mark – first started their activity in Kithituni, they invited Jonathan to the meeting. The story goes that he got up and left at the point where they said that people needed to talk openly about sexual matters. Jonathan was of a generation that simply didn't do this; even though he was clearly, with thirteen children and one wife, a man who probably had something to say on the subject – insights and experience that might prove precious for a generation trying to find guidance on sexual matters.

No. Sex was a private matter. End of discussion.

But Jonathan was unsettled by the meeting. He asked himself: 'How can we not discuss the very thing we need to discuss if we are to stop this pandemic from overwhelming us? What shall I tell these children who are growing up knowing that their parents died of a sexually-transmitted disease, but don't have parents around to teach them?'

Jonathan had an epiphany. One day he stood up in church and announced: 'We have to talk about this disease that is killing us and to do that we must talk about sex.' This change of heart by a septuagenarian who had lived a life of faithful commitment to a woman who has borne thirteen children and who was so respected by the community, spoke as eloquently and effectively as any intervention programme could. If the Church – so central to the life of the community – and its key influencers were able to permit, even encourage, greater openness on matters which, for years, had been taboo, then they had taken a big step towards getting to the root of the thing that had come to destroy them and their neighbours.

But what about the young man or woman who doesn't want to go to church? The people who usually most needed to have the discussion about HIV were often the ones least likely to have it. To engage with them you had to get out 'beyond the gates', just as Rebecca had done in the Kibera – out into the streets, the bars, the markets, the work places. Sooner or later someone had to ask the question, who is my neighbour? And sooner or later a preacher had to preach 'My neighbour is the thinning man who I used to talk to on the way to market; my neighbour is the woman I cut maize with in the *shamba* but who has recently been too ill to work. My neighbour is the sand-boy who spends his money on prostitutes on the Mombasa Highway.'

April's house was close to a poor road that was a tributary of another poor road, which flowed off the main Mombasa highway – itself a poor road. Usually this road was just dust and saw little traffic: people on foot, some on bicycles, and the occasional spastic vehicle. But over the weeks, the dust had been whipped up into great storms by trucks driving down from Nairobi to collect the sand that was being excavated from the dried-up riverbed, and then taking it back to the city to be mixed into concrete by a construction company building hotels, banks and shopping malls there.

The excavation of this riverbed was an environmental disaster in the making; but this quick commerce had other, immediate, consequences. The trucks arrived in the morning and along the road they picked up men and boys to do the digging (they sometimes waved to us from the back of the trucks, clearly euphoric at having been given the employment). They would get paid one hundred Kenyan shillings for twelve hours labour, a pittance that was a princely sum around here. How to turn such wages down? The boys then had money to burn and their new found wealth and energies and lusts made their shopping preferences deadly. If AIDS was a war then the sand-boys were its easily press-ganged recruits.

Late one afternoon, the team went down to see them. We took Mary, the woman who owned Miriam the cow. The team accommodated all ages, both sexes; and the presence of an old woman would give them added respect. These young men would listen to an old woman. We passed through the little conurbation down the road – near where George the Baptist preached – and saw some of the sand-boys not on their shift, in their English Premiere League football shirts, loitering. There were two bars there and the atmosphere was more hostile than in the main town. And there were girls – here, and back in the town, and out on the highway at Sultan Hamud – who were sucking up their wages with their bodies to pay for the food that was failing to grow in their *shambas* from lack of rain.

We walked behind one of the huts that was a shop selling long-life milk, sodas, tomatoes, onions, bananas and mangoes that were in season and keeping people going through the drought. We passed along the track and down to the dried-up River Mikayu that should, in theory, flow on to the Indian Ocean. The waterless river was wide and strangely beautiful and further upstream there were children digging holes, not for sand but for the water that lay a few feet beneath the silt.

In the ground there were heavy tracks and we followed them as they detoured away from the main riverbed, along an offshoot that felt as if it shouldn't be there. The banks of the river were suddenly higher and the tracks bent around out of sight, and it felt like we were in a canyon. And so we were: a truck-made canyon. And as we turned the bend in the 'un-river' there, ahead, were two big trucks waiting to be filled with pay dirt and around them and up on the banks the sand-boys shovelled the sand in with the stamina of men who got paid by the truck load and knew their wages were going to buy them momentary pleasure when the work was done.

They were all stripped to the waist and working in the full glare of the midday sun. I tried to do some digging at their pace but I stopped after five minutes, my chest heaving, to drink some water and retire. I joined Joseph and Johnnie Boy who were talking to some of the resting sand-boys. Joseph had been at school with a few of them. He asked them how much they got paid. Some said 'by the truck'; others said 'by the day'. Joseph then asked the sand-boys what they spent their money on. The furtive laughs and knowing looks gave them away.

Derek, a young man in a Chelsea Football Club shirt, said he was going to use the money to buy a cow with his wages and then sell the milk to support his mother. He said it sincerely but it was clearly a half-wish mixed with an attempt to say what he thought we wanted to hear. He knew who Mary was, that she had a cow, and he knew the boys were from the Church.

Joseph then asked them about HIV/AIDS and what they thought about it. How much they knew about it. They said it was something they were afraid of. They knew about the campaigns for condoms. They'd seen the AIDS posters on the peeling walls of the restaurants in Sultan Hamud. But one, out of bravado, said he didn't care about it and that he was still going to enjoy himself and that if he died he didn't care. 'Say no to Mr Sex posters' weren't going to stop him. His nihilism was a shock but he wasn't that different to any young, English hedonist looking to live for the moment. It's just that in his country the consequences were lethal.

When Joseph asked if any of them knew their status, not one of these young men in this, the most-likely-to-be positive category, said they had taken a test. When he asked them if they'd consider going for a test, the men shook their heads.

They were too afraid to do that.

In this visit to the sand-boys you could see that all things join up and have their interconnections and intersections; that all the tributaries of man's bad choices flowed together and met in this dried-up riverbed, where young men find themselves digging sand for concrete for buildings they'd never see; and that a full truck payload easily leads to a loveless exchange of sweat and blood and semen in a dismal back room somewhere nearby, between people looking to satisfy basic appetites and earn their daily bread.

Whilst On Our Way
Somewhere More Important

Before we set off on this journey many people had said, as if trying to reassure me and maybe themselves, that this trip would be 'a wonderful education for the children'. I don't know what they had in mind: unless going to the funeral of a man who had died from a disease that he had got from having sexual intercourse with someone who was not his wife was what they meant. Was this the extra curricular activity that would compensate for whatever Gabriel might be missing through not being at school? In the morning he would study geography, English and maths with his mother; in the afternoon he would see what can happen to a man who isn't faithful to his wife.

There is no point in hiding death from children; and yet we do all that we can in our culture to keep our dear little ones from knowing that such a thing exists: 'grandpa has gone into the next room'; 'so and so has gone to a better place'; but such sentimental metaphysical puerility simply couldn't be sustained in a culture and society where death – premature, sudden, untimely death – is as expected as sunrise. Most of the children my children played with around our house each day had experienced the loss of a close relative. They had all been to funerals. They had all heard the mournful wailing of mothers, sisters, aunts and grandmothers. In school they sang songs about AIDS: its causes, its consequences, in a way that our own children recite the times tables. 'Take great care…AIDS is a disease…sometimes it is called slim…there is no cure for AIDS…we must take great care…' these poems were their 'Ring A Ring O'Roses', minus the metaphor.

Sooner or later my children were going to see it. Death, the most certain and sure thing we can know, a thing as real and likely as the River Nile being 4,184 miles long or Henry VIIIth having six wives and dying of syphilis, a thing more verifiable than evolution or democracy or quantum physics. It's a fact of life. So why not make it part of our education?

Gabriel and I met the team on the road. The young men – Onesmus, Joseph, Johnnie and George, were all there, as were Catherine and Margaret and two other women I had not met before; it was all part of the organic nature of the response team that anyone could join in at any time: the criteria for qualification: anyone prepared to walk the walk. Also with us for the walk that day was Abednego – Mark's brother, another of Jonathan and Agnes's children. Abednego worked in Sultan Hamud and he was the connection between the team and the man who died. Abednego was himself crippled from childhood polio and he walked with an exaggerated lurch. He had only recently started to join in with the team's activity. A year before he had been lost in a haze of drugs and despair, a despair in part brought on through years of being unable to walk properly. Out of his mind, pushing and dealing ghat and dope for tourists in Mombasa, he was close to ruination before his brother Mark went looking for him and confronted him with making a choice between continuing self-pitying destruction or making a go of his life back in Kithituni. Now, here he was, leading us along the road, walking his mended broken walk, telling us of his plans to sell okra to the supermarkets in Nairobi, showing us the way to a funeral, trying to flag down the transport.

At first, no trucks came – not even the sand trucks taking the excavated riverbed sand back to Nairobi – so we started to walk. It is upon such arbitrary things, such as a passing truck, that an African day turns: the journey could be three hours or twenty minutes depending on being in the right place at the right time; the point is you can't be too pre-planned. Timetables, organisers, diaries, appointments. All the scaffolding that supports the structure of an efficient, purposeful day in the West can't be applied here. 'The thing about Africa is that you must expect nothing,' my godfather had said to me. It was helpful advice.

While we waited Joseph saw a mosquito and he called out: 'Mosquito, mosquito…catch it…kill it…' and everyone played the game, doing the actions: capturing the imagined mosquito with cupped hands and then squashing it by clapping the hands.

As we walk I ask the men questions.

'So, George. Can you think of anything they make in Kenya?'

'The only thing that is made in Kenya, that I can say, is spoons. And on the farming side the thing they make is tea.'

'What about coffee?'

'Yes, we make coffee but we cannot afford the final product that is brought back.'

'I think you are not patriotic, George,' Onesmus said.

'I think you are not patriotic, George,' I said. 'But you are honest.'

We laughed – they laughed – at the paucity of product that comes from their country; and they also laughed at the iniquity, the barefaced ridiculousness of not being able to afford the thing they actually make.

Then they asked me questions.

What do we make in the UK?

I tell them that we don't make very much any more. They ask how this can be when we are so rich. I say it's because we have changed our economy to make money from invisible, intangible things: services, finances, entertainment.

They then ask me how many people have AIDS in the UK I tell them that there are cases but the numbers are not as great as they are here in Kenya. They conclude that people must be more faithful in England. I tell them that statistically we have the highest prevalence of sexually transmitted disease in Europe and have more sexual partners in a lifetime than any other European country. They conclude that people must wear condoms more readily in my country. I'm not sure this is true. I am certain that if I had been a young man living in Africa in the mid 1980s and had my equivalent sexual history I would be dead by now.

Expect nothing. The corollary being 'expect nothing and you will be thrilled when something turns up.' There are sudden cheers as a battered white Datsun pick-up stops to give us a lift. We all pile into the back of it and sit cramped up together with a bag of maize flour and some chickens. As we bump and swerve along the road to Sultan Hamud, we sing songs. They teach me a round: substituting a word – the name of a person – each time: 'Kibaki didn't like it, but Jesus set me free'; repeat... 'BBC didn't like it but Jesus set me free' and then I teach them 'London's Burning' and we are soon screaming out the words 'Fire! Fire! Pour on water! Pour on water!' as our transport skids and slides on the newly muddied road. At the river-crossing the truck actually has to go slow as, for the first time in a long time, there is running water in it; water running down from the hills where last night the rains finally came, late and inadequate, but still appreciated.

Before we reach the junction the truck pulls over to avoid the traffic police seeing that there are twelve people riding in the back. We disembark and walk on and George gives us another weather report.

'Yes. Blessings. Today we are happy. The weather is sunny but, as we can see, there is some wet ground because of last night's rains.'

The Mombasa Road is synonymous with truck drivers and truck drivers are synonymous with casual, passing sex, which is connected to prostitutes that is connected to AIDS. All roads lead to AIDS and this road is the main thoroughfare, the prime filling-station for men's appetites, their loneliness; their need of comfort.

Either side of the road a town of sorts has built up. It consists largely of wooden food stalls and concrete 'hotels' and guesthouses. Behind these are further rows of accommodation, some of it mud and straw; some of it shoddy wood. It is only six miles from the town of Kithituni and yet it is a world away. Here, the community feels transient and the only permanent habitation that exists is here to service 'The Road' and feed the various appetites of the truck drivers.

Ahead of us a big Scania truck pulls up and a man jumps out. In the dust, someone has written 'macho man' with their finger on the rear mud flap and I speculate: He is hungry and tired and he thinks he might stop here for the night. He walks past his truck that is filthy from dust. He checks his pocket for the 'Trust' condoms that he was handed by the American girl who worked for one of those NGOs at Makindu a few hours ago. He doesn't really want to use them but maybe they will bring him luck. It has probably been a while since he has had sex. Because of the big shipments and the lack of good drivers he has not seen his wife – living in Nakuru, some three hundred miles away – for two months. He tells himself that it is not good to go without sex for this long; it is bad for his concentration at the wheel. He knows a girl at the Paradise Lodge Motel – the one who didn't mind him not wearing a condom the last time – and he thinks he'll look for her. Some of the other girls insisted on him wearing a condom, which is annoying. After all who's paying here? But she didn't mind and the extra money will help her get her sister to the secondary school in Kithituni and pay for the okra she dreams of planting in her *shamba* when the rains eventually come.

He paid her extra for not wearing a condom but it was worth it.* She let him do what he liked and she got some pleasure from

---

* In a study of Mexican prostitution, the Berkeley economist Paul Gertler and two co-authors showed that when a client requested sex without a condom, a prostitute was typically paid a 24% premium over her standard fee.

it, too. Afterwards they even had a conversation. They talked about AIDS and they wondered how could something so bad come out of something that felt so good?

Abednego says there is a sick woman we should visit on the way to the funeral and he leads us across the Mombasa road to look for her house. As we cross, skinny cattle are being herded along the edge of the highway. They belong to the Masai and one of their tall, beaded herdsmen drives them nonchalantly across the path of trucks, knowing that they will give way to him. We have seen the Masai herdsmen driving their cattle in search of pastures and last week we read in the newspaper that they had driven their stock into the very centre of Nairobi and onto the lawns of the presidential residence in protest. The lack of rain is driving them to seek even more unlikely pastures, like this truck-stop junction.

We pass behind the first row of buildings and find a dead cow lying across our path that is muddy from the first rain that has fallen here this year. It seems the cow has died because of the drought that has killed the grass upon which they graze. At the next turn we encounter another cow that is a living skeleton. It is so weak and famished that it cannot stand up and it sits there resigned to death. Some of the men decide to help get the cow to its feet. Eight of them gather round the stricken animal and raise him up with a great heave and a cheer. The startled cow stands there, finding his feet and then he moves off to live a little longer.

The woman who was sick lived not far from the track where the dead cow lay, along a path churned up from too much rain too quickly fallen. We had to tightrope along the mud and as we did this Gabriel slipped and stepped into mud that covered his whole foot. Had he been wearing walking boots like mine instead of open sandals this wouldn't have mattered, but the mud clomped to him and there was no immediate way of cleaning it off.

The woman, who was in her fifties, sat on a stool at the entrance to her house which was the simplest type of construction – mud and straw augmented by some broken brick – and too small for us to go inside. We formed a semicircle around her and stood in the mud with our heads in clouds of flies. The flies buzzed around us and little midges – out too early to be mosquitoes – bit at our legs and necks. Even though these were not the malaria-bearing mosquitoes I tried to swat them away from my son with my hat, not wanting to risk him being bitten. I was feeling bad for Gabriel. It wasn't serious but the ordure on his foot, his discomfort, and my inability to do anything about it got to me and I could hear those other voices; not the voices of encouragement but those sceptical voices questioning my reasons for bringing my family on a trip such as this.

The woman was not HIV positive – or at least, she was not sick from AIDS related infections – but she had a cancerous tumour below her breast and she raised her shirt to show us. She said that if she had the money she would pay for an operation but such a thing was beyond her means. Onesmus offered to pray for her as this was all we had to offer and she accepted. After we had prayed for the woman she saw that my son was unhappy. She beckoned him to step forward and with great effort she fetched a container – a gasoline flagon – that held her only water supply. She then asked one of the men to pour the water on Gabriel's leg while she washed off the mud. She was meticulous and wanted to wash his shoes as well. By now everyone was huddled around my son, helping pour the precious liquid, while I lifted him off the ground so that they could clean his sandals. The old woman with the tumour didn't stop until my son's leg and shoes were completely washed clean.

I'd like to think – and did as it was happening – that my son would remember this scene (fitting so tidily into the Biblical: the sick woman washing my son's feet with her precious water) for the rest of his life, but you cannot tell what will sink in. As the scene unfolded I began to realise that this was exactly the kind of experience that would make up for any formal education he might be missing out on by being with me on this trip. The kind of thing you couldn't teach. It felt like a sort of living lesson; it wasn't one I could have set out to find; it was something we stumbled into whilst on our way to something else we thought was more significant. This was the thing we would learn about small acts of kindness: you didn't go looking for them; you simply walked into them.

The funeral took place in an open, almost desert-like tract of land, one side of the Mombasa–Nairobi Railway track. Men and women stood shading themselves beneath umbrellas, waiting for the service to begin. We were not from this community but the gesture of attendance was appreciated by the family of the man who had died. He was a married man, this time with three children. When the service began it was subdued enough for my son to observe: 'Although we're at a funeral there's not that many tears…it seems that they just don't care.'

My son was right about the tears. The service was abbreviated. There were no sentiments expressed at the graveside; no one said this man has gone to a better place; no one said this man will be remembered as a good father or husband; but nor was anyone shedding tears or wailing. It was as if a new, shorter funeral service had been chosen because no one could afford the longer, fuller service, complete with tears and eulogies and wake. This lack of the common expression of grief was, for Onesmus, a deprivation, a consequence of having to do so many funerals. Because of the profligacy of deaths through AIDS there simply wasn't the time or the space to do these things properly any more. It was one of the consequences of AIDS that few people recognised: by numbing reactions at the graveside and truncating the grieving process, it was diminishing the significance of death – and the value of a life. Too much death doesn't necessarily make people healthily aware of the reality; it can actually make them resigned to despair. Once a society stops thinking that death is an insult, an interruption, an end, then death wins. By attending this funeral, the team were not just paying respects to a lost life they were showing disrespect to death. Whilst it was important to accept death as part of life; it was still necessary to rage against the dying of the light.

'Lovin' Human Connection'

I sat in a café belonging to Other Agnes, next to the grain-weigh run by Jonathan and his son Henry, reading the paper, eating a *japati* with sugar and drinking bad instant coffee that I had made myself with the sachet of granules and thermos of hot water provided. If I half closed my eyes I could imagine I was eating pancakes.

There are two national journals in Kenya: *The Standard* and *The Nation*. Every day now, for weeks, these papers had been highly critical of the government and the leadership of Kibaki. The talk was of corruption: a scandal involving a company called Anglo-Irish and the insider-dealing of prominent government ministers. Why, these papers were asking, did Kibaki not sack these ministers; was it, they implied, that he was involved? Kenya was meant to be the fifth most corrupt country in the world. How they calculated this was hard to fathom, but reading about these scandals every day I was starting to believe it myself. What was the source of this corruption: was it a special kind of African corruption that only democracy can wash clean over time? Was it something innate? Or was it a myth chiselled out of racism? (Taffy was a Welshman: Taffy was a thief?) They tell me that in Nigeria (Number 1 in the name of the list survey) corruption is almost in the DNA of the nation now – not just at the highest levels, but out on the streets, in the simplest transactions between brothers. No one could be trusted there and this was what it was becoming like here. I didn't believe it and didn't want to believe it.

The men around me were already eating their lunches of *ugali*, beans, goat stew, chicken, *japati*, rice and *sekuma* (a spinach-like vegetable) and reading the same stories I was. I asked them what they thought about Kibaki. Were the stories true? One man said the stories were being orchestrated by the former leader Daniel Arap Moi – who ruled Kenya for 25 years. Moi, who only a few years ago was pelted with tomatoes at his resignation speech because the people were sick of him, was now a figure of nostalgia for some.

I asked. 'Would it be better if he came back?'

Another man opposite me, mopping his gravy with *ugali* was having none of this.

'No,' he said. 'We can't go back to that Big Boss mentality. The Big Boss mentality is a disaster for Kenya; bad for all of Africa. These men who come to power and then won't let it go. Look at Mugabe in Zimbabwe; look at Museveni in Uganda. We have to move on from this and Kibaki is trying to do that. That is why he is giving his ministers more freedom. It will take time but you will see.'

Further into the paper, there was an article about the launch of American Express RED, rock star Bono and businessman Bobby Shriver's initiative designed to help fight HIV/AIDS. For every pound spent on the card, American Express contributed 1% to the Global Fund. It appeared, with no apparent conscious irony, next to a feature about a woman having the right to choose when she has sex. The piece (judging from the photo) was by a smart, middle-class Kenyan lady. 'I want to sleep with whoever I want, when I want,' she wrote. On the next page there was a recipe tip on how to cook lasagne and spruce up a salad using balsamic vinegar.

At about ten o'clock, Johnnie Boy, Onesmus, Joseph and Georgie-Porgie entered the café and a few minutes later other members of the day's visiting team joined us, including Margaret and Abednego's wife, Catherine, Anton and Oral Roberts. I'd persuaded them to do the brief here instead of in the hot hut with the tin roof and promised to buy them all breakfast – an easy thing for someone like me to do when breakfast for ten can be bought for three pounds. It had taken me a few visits – the funerals and a trip to Makindu – to realise that the young men would have gone a whole day and walked several miles without a meal if I hadn't needed to eat myself and been able to pay their way. They'd survived the last visit by knocking mangoes from the trees. Today we were walking about ten miles and there were no cafés en route.

'Let's eat properly,' I said.

No one refused my offer of breakfast; the 'eat what you can when you can' approach to life meant that when the opportunity was there you took it well. The young men ordered up great piles of *japati* and heaps of scrawny chicken and *sekuma* and rice and while everyone tucked in Onesmus outlined the plan for today: a visit to his uncle Pascal and a woman called Martha. Pascal was HIV positive and for the last few months had been too ill to get to hospital to collect his ARVs (Antiretroviral drugs). Martha had TB and was too scared to take an HIV test even though her TB was almost certainly an AIDS related opportunistic infection and a precursor to full blown symptoms.

I noticed that Onesmus was lightening up. In those first few briefs he'd been a bit stiff; a bit earnest. Earlier, I'd risked insulting him by making a few jokes about the management speak, mimicking him in mock robotic tones: 'I am helping you facilitate your human capacity.' I wasn't sure if the joke had gone down well. But at the end of this little briefing Onesmus put on his hat and his sunglasses and in a self mocking robotic statement said:

'It is time to go. My name is Onesmus, I am lovin' human connection.'

As the ragged fellowship snaked through the Market, Onesmus pointed to the wall where young men sat and watched the world go by. He told me that only a year before this he had been one of those young men sitting, watching the world go by and wearily watching neighbours and relatives die. One day, he had seen the response team pass through the village, much as we were doing now, on their way to see someone who was sick. As they passed, he had asked them what they were doing. They told him and invited him to come and see for himself. He agreed and now here he was.

It was a happy side effect of spending so long getting somewhere that we had time to get to know each other. The walking helped peel away the layers of our lives; got us beyond the jovial front to some of the frustrations we were facing. Joseph was unhappy at not having a job yet; Johnnie Boy wanted to be a journalist; Georgie-Porgie was thinking of being a teacher. Onesmus mentioned his dream of being a doctor. I felt sure (but didn't say) that had any of these intelligent, dedicated, young men been growing up in my country they'd have realised their dreams by now.

Pascal and his wife Rhoda lived a mile out of Kithituni, up a path on the side of a hill overlooking the valley and dried-up River Mikayu. The house was very simple; it was a shed really and someone had painted 'Pentagon HQ' on the side of it. Chickens pecked at grain around a small rondaval and two children stood naked from the waist down in the yard. There was a pall of sickness here and a smell of wood smoke and sweat and something else.

Pascal came to greet us. He was gaunt and moved in slow motion, dressed in a ragged pin stripe suit. We each shook his cold spindly hand and although I knew it was safe to touch I checked my hand afterwards just to make sure I had no grazes. It was easy to see how irrational fear created stigma.

The team had been helping Pascal for a few years, bringing

him food, getting him to hospital for tests and ARVs when they could. Even though they had been supporting him since 2002, and Pascal was familiar with most of the team, he seemed tentative. His wife – who attended the local Salvation Army church when she could – seemed more receptive. She said she was grateful that the church had come to her now that she was too sick to get to church.

Two of the women in the team – Margaret and Catherine – talked and prayed with Rhoda while we talked to Pascal.

'Can I ask how long you and your wife have been unwell?' I asked him.

'Yes, we have been sick for a long time. Since four years.'

'Did the doctor tell you what the problem was?'

'The problem was… Yes. Let me be straightforward with you. When we went to the doctor we got positive. Positive. HIV. That is the disease we are facing in this family. So any assistance you can give. I pray God will bless you.'

'What do you need?'

He said he needed to get to the hospital again. The last time he'd been to the hospital – fifty miles away – his T cell count* was below the two hundred mark. He needed to go back. The ARVs, he said, were not working.

'Is there nothing nearer? No place you can get them?'

'That hospital is where he gets free ARVs,' Onesmus said.

Pascal didn't seem comfortable talking about his condition – why should he? He told me that he was HIV positive but it was a struggle to spell it out. It was a measure of the stigma – the attendant feelings of guilt, failure and despair – that AIDS induced such reticence even in those who were being loved and supported unconditionally. Pascal had never fully come to terms with his

---

* T cells are specialised cells (sometimes called CD4) that protect the body from infection. Most people without HIV have a T cell count of 700-1000. HIV infected people are considered to have 'normal' CD4 counts if the number is above 500. When it falls below 200, you are said to have AIDS.

condition and he seemed embarrassed by it and by extension it was a challenge for him to receive this care and attention, as if he was not worthy of it. Onesmus said it had taken Pascal a few months to realise that whatever he'd done in the past was not relevant to the team coming to help him. Even when there was no judgement people felt judged; such was the power of guilt and shame.

Later, as we set off for Martha's on the next stretch of road, Onesmus was sanguine about his uncle.

'He seemed hopeful. He wasn't despairing. When we saw him last time he was talking about suicide. But he has more hope now.'

'What gives him that hope?' I asked.

'I would say much of this hope is ground on people who have been visiting him. And also ground on faith.'

'You think he has faith?'

'I think he has, but at first because of his status he thought he was not able to have faith. The visits have helped him see that that isn't true.'

Maybe it is easier to attend to the needs of a man in the death throes of HIV/AIDS – to lift his head, hold his hand, wipe his sores, lift him over the pit latrine – than tell that same man he is forgiven for whatever mistakes he made. But maybe, by doing the one, you are doing the other.

We walked on for an hour and a half singing and joking until we arrived at the collection of huts where Martha lived. We sat in a circle around a tree just next to the three huts, a royal delegation for a sick lady, and waited for Martha to come out. Martha emerged from the hut, propping herself on a stick. She was about thirty, quite beautiful, and the deforming sarcoma on her lips were already visible. There was no questioning her condition.

No one could be coerced into taking a test. The teams' approach was that if you cared for people, the care would help them overcome their fear and lead to a change of heart. I was curious to see if it worked.

Martha was visibly moved at being given a visit from ten people, including a *muzungu* from London. Her sister and mother served us all sweet tea and there was much low soft talk and laughter between the team and the family. I remember wondering how I'd feel if this many people spent a whole day coming to see me if I was sick, before realising that in our culture and society – where people were employed or too busy or too socially disconnected – that this would probably not happen.

In the hour the team sat with her talking, laughing and praying, Martha visibly lifted and no longer seemed defined by her disease. This was another aspect of the work that was hard to assess: making people feel like human beings instead of sick victims; and yet getting them to face their true condition. The mission within the mission here – other than extending 'lovin' human connection' – was to encourage Martha to get herself tested.

When Onesmus apologised for not having anything to give her in the way of medicines, Martha said it was good that they hadn't brought a lecture or condoms or even drugs. She was glad that they had brought themselves. She said this gave her enough hope to get herself well, and maybe help others. She said she would like to go for a test now.

It took me a few weeks and a number of visits to understand how this worked. At first, the accepted wisdom of my own world had me calculating whether this was an effective use of time and manpower: I'd ask: 'Shouldn't they be taking this woman drugs or food or something? Shouldn't they be dividing up into three smaller groups? What's the point in making all this effort and walking miles for someone if they're not going to live?'

But going the extra mile was partly the point. I was slow to spot it really – focused as I was on empirical ways of measuring success – but it was these small acts of kindness that were holding things together here. They weren't the added extra, the bonus;

they were it. These people hadn't brought anything because they had nothing to bring but themselves and maybe, in some way, that was enough. After a while I stopped trying to measure the efficiency of these visits and see them for what they were: self-giving, sweaty acts of love.

Major Randive and the Prostitutes

After six weeks of walking to the rhythms of life and death in a rural Kenyan community, we took a giant leap in pace and culture across the ocean to India, where the next wave of the HIV/AIDS pandemic was said to be gathering. We had planned it this way so as to avoid the intolerable heat of India in May. We would return to Kithituni but not before making a journey-within-a-journey that would take us to Mumbai, the Maharastran city of Satara and the far Eastern Indian Province of Mizoram.

Twenty-two years had passed since my wife Nicola and I had been to India. In that time, its population had grown by 350 million, its economic growth was the second fastest in the world (after China); and HIV/AIDS had infected five million of its people. Back in 1985, we were students and our route followed a predictable and hedonistic route. This time there would be no visits to temples or forts; no stoned elephant rides, languishing on lakes; no luxurious and outrageously cheap nights in ex-Maharaja's palaces; instead we would be stopping off in Mumbai, a city with nearly a quarter of a million sex-workers; the indistinct Maharastran town of Satara where people paid to have and watch sex in an open field by a bus station; heading east to the restricted access State of Mizoram, a place dulled and wounded by the opium trade; and then on to the delta city of Calcutta to see what unadulterated poverty and indifference really look like when they conspire.

At least our previous visit prepared us for the shock that is India (something even Africa doesn't do); it prepared us for intolerable heat, probable sickness, the total assault on the senses: oral, aural, olfactory. Despite the country's much trumpeted economic growth, the signs were that the boom was proving as much curse as blessing. 350 million more people made more noise, created more pollution, used more plastic, guzzled more petrol, ate more food, had more diseases and needed more medicine. Despite the daily hagiographies about the Indian economy screened on television and printed in business pages of newspapers and the imminent visit of the American president and the talk of nuclear power, it seemed this boom was unable or unwilling to meet the increased needs of the increasing population.

Nowhere is this dichotomy – the successful accumulation of wealth by the few and the crushing poverty of the many – more conspicuous than in the nation's financial capital, Mumbai. In his book *India: A Wounded Civilization* V. S. Naipaul wrote (in 1977), 'Every day 1500 more people, about 350 families, arrive in Bombay to live. They come mainly from the countryside and they have very little; and in Bombay there isn't room for them. There is hardly room for the people already there.'

Many of these rural families, the would-be Dick Whittingtons who had come to seek their fortune in this city end up in the sex-trade. If in Kenya and Sub-Saharan Africa, the AIDS pandemic had crossed over into the family and become something anyone could acquire; in India the pandemic was thought to be 'contained' within a particular group of people: prostitutes and their clients. In any other country this might seem a manageable grouping; but in India prostitution was on a scale so great that no one was safe from its reach. Mumbai, a city of seventeen million, was said by the Salvation Army to have 200,000 sex-workers. Of those 200,000 most were women. Of those women about 40% were HIV positive (although official statistics are impossible to trust given that a prostitute is the last person going to go for a test).

And of those infected maybe 30% used condoms. Do the maths. Meanwhile, the Indian newspapers all talked of boom.

'Dad, what is a prostitute?'

Agnes, my six-year-old daughter, asked me this as we sat in the back of the black and yellow Fiat taxi on our way to see a drop-off centre for the children of the prostitutes in the heart of Suklajee Road, the official red light area of the city. Ever since we had arrived in Mumbai we had been using this word and sooner or later I was going to have to explain what it meant.

'A prostitute,' I said, trying to modulate an answer appropriate to a six-year-old, 'is someone who sells their body to someone else.'

Agnes seemed satisfied with this description but I knew that it barely did the reality justice. I should have said that a prostitute ('sex-worker' is a less prejudiced and loaded but somehow inadequate term) was someone – almost always a woman – who was so poor and desperate that they were forced to sell their body to someone else because they had no money or work by which to feed themselves. I should have said that those people then had things done to them that they would never have chosen; I should have said that the children she was going to meet were being looked after by the Salvation Army while their mothers were selling their bodies to men and that in this city there were children, the same age as her, who were being used as prostitutes.

Sitting up front, directing the taxi driver through Mumbai's motorised mayhem, sat Nishikant Rananaware, the Project Co-ordinator for the Jeevan Asha project, a ministry that rescues and rehabilitates children caught up in prostitution; helps women get out of sex-work, offers counselling on HIV/AIDS and creates a safe environment for these women and children. Jeevan Asha was named after a Nepalese girl who, at the age of nine, was sold by her father to a woman who trafficked in children. In turn, this woman had sold Asha to a brothel in Mumbai where she was beaten and starved until she submitted to being prostituted. Asha, whose name means 'hope' in Hindi, was one of the few children rescued from her abusers by a local Christian ministry that had decided to do something about it.

It was here, in the back streets of an old colonial city, the gateway and back door of the old British Empire that the Salvation Army were doing what they had always done: ministering to the prostitutes. Whether he knew it or not Nishikant was doing the work that William Booth and his Slum Sisters had started 150 years before in the shack slums of London, ministering to the women and children caught in the trap of prostitution. The scale of the problem in Mumbai was greater but the nature and causes of these abuses were really no different and the outcome just as abject: Booth could have been describing some of the children of Mumbai when he wrote in his book: 'thousands upon thousands of these poor wretches are not so much born into this world as damned into it. The bastard of a harlot, born in a brothel, suckled on gin, and familiar from earliest infancy with all the bestialities of debauch, violated before she was twelve, and driven out into the streets by her mother a year or two later, what chance is there for such a girl in this world…yet such a case is not exceptional. There are many such differing in detail, but in essentials the same. And with boys it is almost as bad…'

In fact, for boys in Mumbai it was worse for there was greater demand for girls and this meant mothers would keep their girls for sex-work whilst abandoning their sons to fend for themselves. When we arrived at the drop-off centre, most of the children there were boys.

The taxi dropped us off at the edge of Suklajee Road and from there we walked up a narrow street of two-storey stores on one side; one-storey shacks on the other. Nishikant had rented a space for the drop-off centre in one of these two-storey properties and he had chosen his site well: this was the business district, the hub and factory floor of the sex-work industry. The street had the hum and hubbub of a bazaar; women lay on beds outside the shacks all along this road; old men did their ablutions standing in mud amongst poultry. It was the usual theatre of the bungled and the botched, a pageant of poverty that is so much a part of India's image it seems acceptable.

Nishikant led us to the 'centre' – a small room turned into an office, with computer and a kettle, some chairs for people to wait and rest or receive counselling. And then there was an upper floor, a half attic really, where the children of the sex-workers would sit and receive some education, a little food and play games. This room could only be reached by ladder and its ceiling was too low for a grown man to stand but when we looked there were eight boys sitting up there cross legged laughing and smiling at the sudden attention they were getting. These Jeevan Asha boys, squashed into a room the size of my bathroom for hours every day, were the lucky ones. Somewhere, in another part of the city where there was no drop-off centre, children this age were sitting – more likely lying – drugged up on pills so that they would sleep while their mothers serviced their clients. And in another street not far away from here there was a building where young girls and boys were incarcerated for the purpose of having sex.

'Now I will take you to see where the prostitution happens,' Nishikant said. 'It is better if your children stay here and you must be careful to take photographs.'

The red light area is effectively seven or eight blocks running perpendicular to Suklajee Road. Whatever squalor I had seen so far on this journey was but a prelude to the scenes that Nishikant was about to show me. He had warned me to be careful about taking pictures, partly out of respect for privacy, but more out of deference to the pimps who controlled the activity here. Mindful of his instruction, I held my camera at arms-length as if just walking and then snapped the shutter, hoping something might come out.

'This building here is full of eunuchs.' Nishikant pointed to the building on our right. Three storeys high, with little balconies covered in colourful, drying laundry, there was no sign of any activity.

'And that building over there is where they keep children for sex. But we cannot go there. It is not safe.'

'What about the police? Don't they try and stop it?'

Nishikant said that the police did not come here.

The Alexander cinema had a massive poster advertising the classic Bollywood movie *Chacha Bhatija* sitting atop its roof. In the poster, corpulent, clean, smooth skinned Indians posed in fine clothes and romantic embraces. (Bollywood had its own underclass of people who had sold themselves to get into the industry.) Nishikant said that the cinema also showed pornographic movies which fuelled the appetite: people would leave the cinema, their blood up, and seek gratification in the brothels off Suklajee Road.

He then led me across the street to an alley way and a side entrance to another building.

'Here is brothel,' he said.

I don't know why I was surprised at the depravity of what we stepped into. Maybe it is because, for some reason, brothels and the activity within them have gained some level of credence, even glamour, through literature and poetry and film and art; after all 'it's the oldest profession in the world', people sometimes say by way of condoning it; with some colourful, famous antecedents and practitioners. Perhaps it was these glamorised memories, a kind of amalgam of Mata Hari, Toulouse Lautrec and Dodge City bar-room saloons that made me expectant of lace, perfume, some kind of cabaret. But this was no house of mirth, no palace of delights. It was a house where the pathetic endgame of desire and abuse meet and play themselves out. The smell of drains might have been a coincidence – but it added to the sense of ruination. We entered into immediate dark and it never got any lighter. A staircase climbed up into the bowels of this building and at the top we found a corridor with corrugated tin walls with doors either side. At the other end of the corridor a child – a boy maybe the same age as my son – sat staring at nothing in particular while in the room behind him a man (from where do they all come?) did things to the boy's mother for the price of a loaf of bread.

Nishikant led me along the corridor to a room where an elderly woman – a Madam – sat nursing a two-week-old baby that belonged to one of her working girls. I'm not sure what started me crying: the sight of the boy sitting outside his mother's deadening bed, or this baby and the old woman, suddenly smiling as she recognised Nishikant. I was embarrassed by my tears but Nishikant touched my shoulder and steadied me, nodding, almost grateful for my reaction. The woman went to get two other Madams – I presumed they were Madams from their ages – and we all of us stood in this room, the baby lying asleep in the small patch of light that came in through the hole in the wall. The women were all happy to see Nishikant and expectant of something. They wanted Nishikant to pray and he asked me if I would like to. I remembered another piece of advice Ian Campbell had given me. 'Don't think you have anything to take into these situations. Remember, God is already there, at work; you just walk into the activity of the kingdom.' My prayer was short and to the point. Desperation keeps a prayer terse and focused.

I asked if I could take a photograph and the woman obliged me. The Indian genius for dishing up colourful, photogenic squalor for photographers was still unmatched. But as I stopped to take a picture of this scene, fancying in it something real, something salutary, I recalled another picture I had once taken of an Indian woman over twenty years before. That photograph hangs on the wall of my house in London. I had been walking around the *Arabian Nights*-like town of Jaisalmeer, Rajasthan, when I saw a woman in the window of her own house, sipping tea from a saucer, her beautiful lined face and hooked aquiline features perfectly framed by the wood and whitewash window. She never saw me. But she's been on my wall for twenty years at home and I had always told myself that it was my brush with the simple beauty of the poor. But now, as I took this picture, I wasn't thinking about blowing it up some day and hanging it for show; but I pictured myself showing it to someone and saying 'Look, this is a brothel and that is a two-week-old baby and that is a Madam and please don't say what a great photograph; say instead, what an appalling scene; what combination of events has to occur to construct a scene as desperate as that?'

That was the question that started to rattle inside my head. Because after the tears comes the anger (although you have to think about who or what to direct that anger at). If there are 200,000 sex-workers in Mumbai then there at least 200,000 clients. Why are there so many? And if, as is the case here and all over the world, most of the clients are men, then someone has to ask why are so many men seeking gratification in this way? What is happening, or not happening, that they will risk disease and the degradation of another human being for ten minutes (the average time spent with a prostitute) of sex with a stranger? Is there really no alternative? Is the intimacy – the true intimacy they desire and that we are wired to enjoy – impossible to find? What is behind this endemic – pandemic – of sexual dysfunction? Too many people? Not enough women? Bad education? A distortion of sex? Abuse? Lust? Not enough committed marriages? What? Because economics only explains one half of this problem – the question of why so many women are driven to prostitution; it doesn't explain why the men, with the money in their pockets, choose to spend it this way.

The train took a long time to pass out of Mumbai. The city – officially fourteen million people, unofficially closer to seventeen million – spread, like so many cities, beyond its capacity, bulging with the hopeful, the homeless, the displaced, all drawn to the metropolis for a thousand different reasons and the same reason: the promise of a better life and the rumour of boom. We sat in first class, air-conditioned and cushioned, amongst the most likely beneficiaries of this economic upsurge. Many of them sat reading newspapers and business magazines that repeated back the re-enforcing mantra: 'India is booming.'

In a commercial break on the BBC World television news programme we had seen an advertisement for a new town, set amongst palm trees and gardens and waterfalls, with accommodation like holiday chalets and endorsed by Western celebrities. It was a slick advertisement and the place – all glass and shining metal – was a hybrid Eastern paradise crossed with Western pragmatism, like the result of a cross fertilisation between Milton Keynes and Phuket. As the train pulled away from Mumbai and the landscape flattened out to fields and the building-work thinned I looked out for this new paradise (the advertisement had never said where it was) but it never appeared. Instead the scene went from urban dilapidation to impoverished countryside with no suburban in between.

Our next destination was the Maharastran town of Satara. Satara was a fair barometer of the Indian situation: caught somewhere between rapid growth and messy squalor. It had no temples or sites of note but it was famous for being a town of ill-repute and its reputation made it a kind of junction of vice. It was here – in this modern day Gomorrah – that we met a genuine saint.

Major Randive was an unlikely hero; but perhaps unlikeliness is a necessary, even essential, criteria for true heroism. He met us at Pune train station and because of his bespectacled, plain, rotund appearance I barely registered him. His more conspicuous colleague – Pravin – (the Indian equivalent of an Onesmus back in Kithituni: that is, a volunteer in communal response; affiliated with the Salvation Army but not a member) – wore a woollen Nehru jacket and thick Rajasthan-style moustache and insisted on carrying our bags. In the car, Randive was quiet and I sensed he was hesitant at having this British family turn up in his town and worried at having to put on a good show; Pravin was formal and talked somewhat stiffly of the 'programme' we were to see, using the same jargon I had heard in the response team in Kithituni. As I sat in the back of the car my heart sank; I had the same sensation I had had when I first met the team in Kenya: Is this it? Is this the response to the problem of HIV/AIDS here: a bag of insecurities and small fat man in glasses?

This feeling of defeat deepened as we entered the indistinct ugliness of Satara. Mumbai had been exciting because it was appalling; Satara had no depraved glamour to get the adrenaline going. It is somehow more bearable to visit a slum in a major conurbation than the middling squalor of a mid-sized city. Mumbai and Calcutta have the frisson of excitement, a buzz, which counters the degradation, at least for a time. But then maybe this was the kind of place where truly selfless heroes lived; it was harder to live in this unappealing, not-quite-awfulness than in the obviously dynamic and heroic degradation of the big cities.

Satara was renowned for one thing: a field where people went to have sex and/or watch people having sex. (They usually ended up doing both, the one leading to the other; the field operating as a kind of teaser commercial.) People would travel to Satara from over a hundred miles away to see it. The startling thing about this activity was that it didn't take place somewhere out of the way; the field was in the very heart of the city. It was bordered by the main road on one side and a bus station on the other. A wall about a foot high provided a perimeter that doubled as a viewing point. Every night, at about nine o'clock, men would gather here in the dark and stand on the wall. The field was partially lit by the light thrown from the market stall but it was mostly gloom in which it was just possible to make out the shadow-figures of couples copulating. Prostitutes would loiter at the wall's edge where the young men were stretching up on tiptoe and peering in an effort to see something. Having found a client from these tiptoeing young men they would then lead them out into the field where they would lay down a newspaper as a bed upon which to have intercourse. Bolder viewers would walk right out into the field and stand right next to the couples having sex. Sometimes couples had to shoo away the stray dogs which hung around in packs and lived by the refuse dumps behind the bus station.

The Major described all this to me but I did not believe it happened in quite so brazen a fashion.

'Tonight I will take you to the prostitution area,' he said. 'And you will see the field where the people they are making the sex. But we must be careful. I cannot go in my uniform and you must not use your recorder. I have my contacts there. Maybe they can help you interview with a prostitute there. But we must be very careful.'

After dinner, Randive went to change into his plain clothes get-up. It would not look good for a Salvation Army officer to be seen near the field at night. When he reappeared he looked even more suspicious in black bobble hat and jacket; Pravin was no less a sore thumb in his hat and gloves. Timothy – a local man who was part of the Major's AIDS response team also saw fit to wear a woollen hat. I had no reputation to protect and went as I was. The four of us set off into the night, laughing at each other's poor disguises and apprehensive of what we might see.

When we arrived the field was empty but for stray dogs loping in the darkness. There were some young men standing on the wall laughing and joking, geeing each other up to step off the wall and take a prostitute out into the gloom. A few women in saris huddled in groups near the wall. There was a bustle of people walking to and fro but the show had not yet started.

Randive wanted to find out how much we would have to pay if we wanted to have sex in the field. He walked the perimeter of the wall until he found a woman – maybe in her thirties – standing, waiting to be approached. She did little to make herself more alluring (if that's the word). She wore a purple sari and her face and arms were heavily decorated with henna stains. There was a younger woman with her who turned out to be her daughter of fourteen years old. Randive did his best impression of an interested punter and asked her how much. 300 rupees (£4) to go with her; 150 rupees to go with her daughter. Either fee was enough to feed them for a week. He thanked her and walked away.

Business was proving slow on this night. So far, only one man had stepped off the watching wall and into the murk with one of the women who stood, just a few feet into the field, coaxing men to join them. We watched him follow her with her *Times of India* mattress out into the field and pick a spot some fifty yards away where there was some privacy. He was about 25 years old and his friends on the wall were laughing and cheering at his sheepish form disappearing into the gloom; the young man seemed to be acting out of some need to prove himself, to dare to take a risk by going with a prostitute in the famous Satara Sex Field.

And what a risk. This man was probably expecting to contract little more than some minor STD − if indeed he was even thinking that at all; but his watching friends might as well have been cheering him to an untimely and agonising death. There was an 80% chance that man would not put on a condom. There was a 20% chance the woman he was about to lie with was HIV positive.

Awareness of HIV/AIDS and its dangers isn't great in India. The wave of AIDS hasn't crashed here yet; it is still building − through the deadly double tidal flows of the sex industry and the increasing number of truck drivers stopping off in towns like Satara, carrying the freight of India's boom to and from the cities. The problem is on such a massive scale that UN agencies have concluded that India will become the world centre of the disease in the next decade. And yet the National Aids Control Organisation (NACO), which coordinates the Indian government's response to the spread of the disease, has routinely dismissed UN estimates on HIV/AIDS, stressing that India remains a low-prevalence country.

This dismissive attitude was evident on the ground. Randive approached two men who were loitering, building up the courage or whatever it took to find themselves a prostitute. Pretending to be a pimp he asked them if they were looking for girls. At first they said they were not here for girls but were just curious to see what was happening. One of the men said he was looking for his sister. She had, allegedly, run away from her husband who was abusing her and had taken refuge in one of the brothels in Satara. This was a common enough story in India but Randive said he would ask the Madams if they knew about this girl. The man wrote down her name on a piece of card.

Randive knew most of the Madams in town; for four years he had been trying to persuade them to let the children of their sex-workers attend his little school that was next to his house and part of the Salvation Army compound. The Major had high expectations for the children; he had offered to pick them up in a bus (he didn't have it yet) and provide them with an education as well as respite from being exposed to their mother's work. Like all real saints, Randive was a pragmatist. If you can't stop the prostitutes then at least help their children, even if this means the prostitutes paying for their children to attend school with money made from selling their bodies. Booth himself had been quick to separate the vice of prostitution from the person caught in the trap of having to sell their body: 'when, however, we cease to regard this vice from the point of view of morality and religion, and look at it solely as a factor in the social problem, the word prostitution is less objectionable. For the social burden of this vice is born entirely by women.'

The other man said he was thinking about going with one of the girls in the field. When Pravin asked him if he was afraid of catching AIDS, the man said he did not care about it. He did not really believe he would catch it. As with governments, so with individuals: if it didn't suit them to believe the evidence they dismissed it.

Pravin said there was a good chance he would get infected, especially if he didn't use a condom. The man said even if he did, he still didn't care. He was showing bravado, but there was a nihilism in him too, not unlike the sand-boy in Kithituni. It was a spirit of 'so what?' that came as much out of hopelessness as ignorance.

Randive had said he'd try and fix an interview with one of the Madams for me. He led me away from the field and out across the main street where an old long-wheel base Land Rover was parked and a handsome driver sat reading a newspaper spread open on the steering wheel. Randive and the man clearly knew each other and we were invited to jump in the back. The man was an ex-policeman who had become a chauffeur for sex-workers, driving them in from towns as far as one hundred miles away. I sat there while the Major and the ex-policeman chatted in Marathi. The man then went off and returned a short time later with a short, wiry, strong looking woman, maybe fifty years old. She joined us in the very back of the Land Rover. Randive introduced her as a Madam; many of her girls were out in the field, although tonight she said work was slow because the police were doing one of their sporadic clampdowns. Randive said she was happy for me to ask her about her work – HIV/AIDS in particular. He translated. She was clipped and fidgety throughout our discussion. I asked her about HIV/AIDS and the effect it was having on her work. Her impression was that the work was suffering because of fear about the disease. What about condoms? She said the girls – at least her girls – all insisted on using them and refused sex with men who wouldn't wear one; but I instinctively felt she was just saying this for my benefit. She and other Madams were part of a local AIDS awareness programme that distributed information leaflets to sex-workers. It was hard not to think they went through the motions of receiving and distributing these leaflets to appease the government. That way the government looked like it was doing its job, and they could carry on doing theirs. I asked her if her girls went to the hospital for testing but she said this was hard for them do to. Of course it was. What prostitute would want to know or even declare her status? I was beginning to see what Randive had told me: that there was no real way of knowing the prevalence rates of HIV in India when most of those infected were the group of people least likely to declare their status for fear of losing their livelihood. It took an engagement slightly more radical than handing out information to change this.

Just before she went, Randive asked the Madam if she knew of a girl (he showed her the name on the card) who had run away from her husband and was hiding out in one of the brothels here in Satara. She nodded immediately. Yes. The girl was staying with her. Randive asked her if she was doing sex-work. The Madam said she wasn't and that she did not want to let her do it. The girls would support her and try and get her money to return home to her husband. The trouble is the girl did not want to go back because she feared being beaten. Randive said he would help find somewhere for the girl to live. The Madam thanked him and left.

Call it a blessed connectedness, serendipity or blind chance. For me it showed something very important – and fairly marvellous – about Randive: he was connected and his connectedness was a natural consequence of his lack of fear and prejudice and a willingness to serve others.

Major Randive lived with his wife Ratnamala and their fifteen-year-old daughter Priyanka on the Salvation Army compound that consisted of a church, a school building and a house. Their accommodation was humble and too small to put up a visiting family like us. Anticipating this the Major had reserved a room in a nearby hotel – 'de Luxe' – and this was to be base for our stay in Satara. The 'de Luxe' was symbolic of India's current self-image: that of a wannabe superpower with a credibility problem. It reeked of aspiration and with its marble floors and fountain and chandeliers and porcelain lavatories it temporarily impressed a tired family who had grown used to pit latrines and power for only three hours a day back in Kenya. The credibility gap soon appeared: room service plates and cutlery piling up unwashed just outside our door, no water at certain hours of the day, grime edging the tiles of the bathroom. All liveable with and not exactly bringing hardship; but somehow more obvious, and exacerbated by the pretension; they were promising something they couldn't deliver. This kind of pretension is harder to take in a country of 260 million living on less than a dollar a day, where one thousand children die of diarrhoea every day; and yet it is everywhere: adverts with glamorous couples living in outsized Spanish style villas stuffed with household appliances, unaffordable to the masses. And newspapers producing a flow of uninterrupted good news about the improving economy and higher living standards for all. Meanwhile in Satara – surely a better barometer of whether things were improving than the mega metropolis – thousands of women and girls still had to sell themselves because they could not earn a living.

I put this to Major Randive at dinner. Do you think things are getting better for the poorest people in India?

He said it was hard to think so when many people in this town did not even have a roof over their heads.

Randive was not political. He didn't sit around abstracting about what the government should do when there was so much to be getting on with. But he was saddened by the situation in Satara – and out in the larger district of Maharastra, where flooding in the last few years had wrecked people's lives.

'When they had the floods you only heard about Bombay. No one mentioned what happened in the countryside.'

As a Major in the Salvation Army he had a salary which gave him some measure of security. His family had somewhere to live and they had enough money to eat well. But life was a struggle for most of the people he served. Here, in India, incomes were higher than in Kenya, but so were the costs. Randive had a large 'parish' to pastor. He had no vehicle of his own (we were paying for the jeep for the duration of our stay) except a Honda Hero motorbike; getting to some of the more remote villages was hard for him. Even if he had had a vehicle the cost of fuel was prohibitive. He had a small team of volunteers who were helping him with the HIV/AIDS response work, but they too had families and the money he gave them was inadequate.

Pravin was married with a child. He had travelled from the city of Abedneggar some three hundred miles away to be here. He had no income at all (as far as I could tell) and this tension was obviously wearing him down. He worked part-time at a hospital in his home city, but he also worked for the Salvation Army regional response team. Neither paid him sufficient to feed his family; his wife was having to work as a nurse, which meant leaving their child with her parents. Pravin had not seen his wife for a month and his daughter for two. He was like so many of his countrymen: an itinerant hopeful, having to sacrifice any semblance of stable family life in order to earn a living which never materialised.

Major Randive had a lot on his mind and a lot in his hands. He was a juggler. Juggling his responsibilities to a 'parish' which took in a vast region and contained a microcosm of worldly problems, each of them enough in themselves to overwhelm. He wanted to show us as much as he could and had hired a vehicle for us to visit the villages where there had been catastrophic flooding the year before (an event I remember being reported in our news as floods in Mumbai). If Randive was a shepherd, he was one of those shepherds with a far-ranging herd and he was prepared to go a long way in the care of his flock, even for the one or two strays.

He took us to two villages some four hours drive from Satara. On the way we were stopped by road-police twice. Both times they asked to look at our passes and both times they asked for money. Randive's uniform gave him some authority and he showed them his Salvation Army papers. I sat in the back, refusing to pay a single rupee. I told Randive to tell them I was a BBC reporter looking into the phenomenon of petty corruption among road police in India (a documentary you could make in pretty much any country we visited on this journey). The letters BBC seemed to have some clout. They waved us through, smiling and apologising for any inconvenience they might have caused.

After three hours we reached the first village in the district of Kohlapur. Kothali was largely Christian. It had a church (not Salvation Army, but Pentecostal) and most of the population worked the land. We could still see evidence of flood damage all around. The houses, like the houses in the village in Kenya, were largely made from mud and wood. In Kenya the villagers were suffering from lack of rain; here they were battling the opposite. In both places I asked the question about the weather changing and in both places I got essentially the same answers: drought and flood were not in themselves the surprise; it was the timing and intensity that was alarming; the predictable was getting harder to predict.

Randive and a team of helpers had come here a few months before to help rebuild many of the houses; we could still see gaps like bomb blasts where the rising waters had pushed though the flimsy mud and wood of the homes. There was also a clear 'tide mark' on the side of the houses – about the height of a man's shoulder – showing how high the flood waters had got. Many houses were empty. It was catastrophes like these that were fragmenting life and driving whole communities to the city in search of another new one.

A young man called Timothy had travelled with us on this

journey. Timothy was from Satara and he had been assisting the over-stretched Major in the AIDS response work. In Satara Timothy had befriended a former sex-worker who was now an integral part of Randive's team (although team makes it sound more organised than it was).

Timothy had likewise identified a number of young people in the village – including a young couple – as being potential helpers in communal response. The man and wife were both HIV positive. The story seemed to be that the man had got infected by sleeping with a prostitute some years before whilst on a trip to the city in search of work. After failing to get a job, he had returned to the village and now his wife was infected.

Timothy led us to their home which was like most homes we had seen: dark, furniture-less, but with bright, clean stainless steel stacked pots and pans proudly arrayed like some proof of cleanliness and victory over the oppressive muck and disease all around. This couple also had a son, aged nine, who was HIV positive. Despite their situation the couple's warmth and friendliness was striking. They did not seem hopeless at all. After discovering that he was HIV positive the man had almost killed himself; but his wife, a Christian, had persuaded him to live and he himself had converted. Rather than sink into despair and perhaps death, they were both trying to make something of their lives; openly talking of their status and playing a role in educating their community as to the dangers of HIV/AIDS. Despair was a common cause of death in India and suicide more commonplace than statistics suggest. Hope – the obvious antidote to despair – was not something easy to manufacture or conjure. But this couple's outlook was not the fatalism that seemed to infect many of their countrymen. I say infect because fatalism (what will be will be; it is our lot; or even punishment for actions in a past life etc) is a kind of destructive disease in and of itself and tends to foster indifference and inaction wherever its prevalence is high. Hope, expressed in the from of an active, practical loving connection, extended from one person to another, made a very big difference in the lives of those who had it.

The village of Malwadi was some sixty kilometres away, in the district of Sangli. Malwadi was a collection of houses around a set of stables, with the animals in the midst of the living quarters. The people had no church building, but it was Randive's hope to raise enough money to build something that might double as community centre and church meeting place. (The amount of hoping-for-things-not-yet-seen this man did was breathtaking.)

It was a Sunday and the people were expectant of a service. Randive asked me if I would preach.

'About what?'

'About anything you like. After that I will talk to them about AIDS. And whatever else we need to discuss.'

Nicola and I and the children were led to someone's house and offered floor on which to sit. We were then served *chai* and offered light food which we declined as we had already been fed in the last village – a delicious, simple lunch of *dhal* and rice and *chapatti*.

As I sat there, brushing flies away and wondering what on earth I would say for a sermon, the community started building a church in the yard. They took a plank of wood and laid it down with a tree trunk at each end. They took a tarpaulin and laid it on the wet ground. They made a sort of alter from a table. Then people gathered in a semicircle. We – 'the visiting dignitaries' – were offered the only chairs. Randive and two of the men from the village formed a band and sat cross-legged on the ground by the stable. A *tabla* was brought out and handed to Randive who started to drum it with some skill. The man next to him had what looked like a one-string sitar, if such a thing exists. The third man was the singer.

The service (not really the right word) began with the third man singing a plaintiff, yearning hymn which Pravin translated as meaning 'there are no gods like you'. In a land where there are many gods jockeying for pre-eminence, these words were a bold statement and, possibly, a dangerous one. I wondered what it was about this God – the God of Christian tradition – that was so exceptional to them? These people had grown up with many gods; they had most likely tried other gods. They were probably better placed to make a comparison and fair assessment. How had they come to this statement?

Randive dabbed the skins of the *tabla* and sang backing without any self-consciousness while the homemade sitar player extracted a sound from his one-stringed instrument that was so rich it was hard to account for. The congregation (not really the right word either) had now grown to about eighty people and some of them joined in with the words which continued describing the attributes of this most singular God. We were sitting in a farmyard with animals all around us. Two cows were eating hay from a manger. Three Eastern men were offering worship. People – some of them shepherds – were dressed in simple tunics. A mother was nursing an infant.

A faded picture of William Booth, the founder of the Salvation Army, hung on the wall of the church hall. With his Levantine features and beard reaching down to his sternum Booth looked like an Old Testament prophet. I had seen this portrait in the drop-off centre in Mumbai, and in the HIV testing rooms there; as well as in the Commissioner's office in Nairobi and I would encounter it again in other countries. Indians liked to put portraits of their heroes and gods on their walls (Ganesh, the elephant god, next to a picture of Jesus, next to a picture of Ghandi, next to a picture of Sachin Tendulkar the great cricketer or Manmohan Singh, the current prime minister). But this picture of Booth was on its own. And it always seemed incongruous. This portrait seemed to be the official one, like that portrait of Queen Victoria (Empress of India – a country she never visited) looking like she was wearing twenty petticoats. Booth's own picture had outlasted those of the Kings and Queens whose portraits had been taken down in India over half a century ago. Where the British monarchs were a part of history, Booth still commanded a reverence, as though he were an active presence. It is possible to see Booth and his army as a kind of relic of Empire; but that description really can't explain his Church's continued acceptance and success in places like Satara.

India was the Salvation Army's oldest mission field and it was first trod by a certain Frederick Latour Tucker of the Indian Civil Service, who, after reading a copy of the *War Cry* (the Salvation Army's weekly journal) became a Salvationist and, as Major Tucker (later Commissioner Booth-Tucker), took the Indian name of Fakir Singh and commenced Army work in Bombay on 19th September 1882. Unlike other missionaries of the day, Tucker and his soldiers adopted Indian food, dress, names and customs and gained ready access to the people, especially in the villages. In addition to evangelistic work, they started social programmes for the relief of distress from famine, flood and epidemic. Educational facilities such as elementary, secondary and industrial schools, cottage industries and settlements, were provided for the 'depressed classes'.

A bearded, middle-aged man, wearing the wrap-nappy style loin cloth, was putting up his HIV/AIDS educational charts on the wall next to the portrait, ready for the community conversation that Randive and his team were facilitating. I wanted to make sure the man knew who the man on the wall was.

'Can you tell me who that is?' I asked.

'That is William Booth. He is a great man. He helped the poor all over the world. And the Salvation Army are helping us today.'

All morning we had moved through the slum area of Koregaon, not far from Satara. Families of four, five, six, were sharing 'accommodation' the size of an Englishman's garden shed. Unlike most garden sheds, these sheds did not have power. Randive held a quick meeting in the largest home where about twenty of us crammed in to talk about HIV/AIDS. A quarter of the young men present volunteered to help with the response in their community where there were many people infected. They had a programme of collecting waste and the money from this was being used to help support those families affected by the disease.

Koregaon had a 'red-light' area although there was insufficient power to electrify neon lights at night. Local men didn't need any guiding lights to find what they wanted: they just walked down to the row of corrugated tin front houses that ran parallel to the sewage drain. Randive led us to one of these houses. It was essentially a two-room structure with attenuated outhouses or 'stables' in which the women serviced the visitors.

It was just after noon and business would be slow enough for us to talk to the Madams and maybe the prostitutes, too. Randive had been targeting this brothel for the last four years, hoping to persuade the Madams to let him take the children of their prostitutes to his school during the day. It seemed a reasonable offer, but it would mean the workers paying something out of their wages for their children to attend the school, which would of course mean the Madams paying.

The Madams were expecting us. They seemed delighted and amused at having a British family under their roof and for the first few minutes we were an ethnic sensation. They made us all tea and giggled at the sight of my wife and daughter's blond hair, their fair skin. The Madams were easy to identify as they were all of them over sixty and somehow more at ease than their workers. The prostitutes – six of them – sat with us, fidgeting. One of them, a beautiful and open-faced girl of fifteen, sat on her haunches, her stunning face resting in her painted palms. Another prostitute sat crouched in the corner holding a child of maybe three or four years old. This woman wanted my daughter to sit on her lap; suddenly she grabbed roughly at Agnes's wrist and pulled her towards her. My daughter is strong and she resisted. I expected the woman to respect Agnes's wishes but she ignored them and continued to pull. In the end my wife interjected: 'It's okay. I think she doesn't want to.' The woman finally let go. It was a fleeting incident, but in that sudden grab you could detect the response of a woman who had been abused for so long she'd lost a physical sensitivity.

Randive was a canny operator. This visit had a double purpose. One: 'Show Brook the prostitution area and the efforts of the Madams to "educate" their staff as to the dangers of HIV/AIDS.' Two: 'Use the presence of Brook and his family to get the Madams to agree to his offer of letting the children of their workers go to his school.' Several children aged between one and ten were with us in the room and Randive sat one of these children on his knee and repeated his offer to the Madams, using me as a kind of collateral: 'Brook is trying to see the work we are all doing with HIV/ AIDS. He knows about my school. Tell him what you are doing.'

The Madam produced an information leaflet about AIDS, as well as a folder, illustrating different kinds of sexually transmitted disease. It was a graphic book picturing the stomach churning effects of having unprotected sex with multiple partners; they passed it around as though it were a coffee table book picturing the latest fashion accessories. The Madam explained that these information packs were being distributed by another Madam (the one I had met in the Land Rover) and that they were very aware of the dangers of HIV/AIDS. The Madams were spearheading AIDS response, which was not entirely helpful to their livelihoods: greater awareness (fear of AIDS) meant less work for them, which in turn meant less money.

A knock interrupted the conversation. A man, maybe 25 years old, stood outside the entrance, looking anywhere but at us. One of the Madams motioned him to walk round the back and she went through the door to meet him (I could see them through the gap in the wall). He handed her the money up front and then she came back and asked the beautiful girl with the painted palms to attend to him. The girl seemed slightly disappointed, she had been listening to the conversation carefully; but now she had to get to work. She stood up and nodded to us and then went through the flimsy door and into one of the adjoining 'stables'.

'How much did he pay you?' I asked the Madam.

'Twenty rupees.' (About £2.50.)

'How long will that man get with her?' I asked.

'Fifteen minutes.'

The next fifteen minutes went by very slowly as I tried not to think about what was happening the other side of the corrugated tin wall. I asked them how many clients a day they went with. Four of five was about average. And did they use condoms?

'If the customer doesn't allow us we don't do the sex.'

The Madam said this slightly mechanically; it seemed said for my benefit.

'Did they like their work?'

The Madam explained that they did it because they had to. And if there were alternatives they would take them. But around here there was no other work and they would starve without this income. My thoughts kept drifting through the tin wall. I thought I could hear noises from next door.

'Why do so many men want to have sex with prostitutes?' I asked.

The Madams and the girls smiled. They seemed relieved. With all this focus on them and their work it was good to talk about the issue: not the issue of supply; the deeper, more difficult issue of demand.

'Is it that they can't have sex elsewhere?'

'That man in there is married,' the Madam said.

'So what's the problem?'

She smiled.

'Men. They cannot control themselves.'

Paneer returned from having had sex with the man who I

could see skulking away, back to whatever it was he did. She was now self-conscious and sat slightly back, in the shadows, wiping her mouth and redoing her hair which was held up with a plastic flower pin.

Randive still had the child sitting on his knee.

'Would you like to come to my school?' he asked the boy.

The boy nodded, hardly believing it.

The Madam suddenly announced that they would like to pay for the children to go to the Major's school. Randive looked quite overcome at this spontaneous decision – a decision he had spent the last four years hoping and praying for. In response he offered up a prayer. We all bowed our heads and Randive thanked God for these women and their children. How natural it seemed to ask God's blessing on this communion of the abused; but then, as he later told me, Randive was following a God who had hung out with a prostitute, healed and put 'in a right way'. 'It is our pleasure,' he said, 'to work for a God who loved everyone.'

All Randive had to do now was get the Madam 'of the field' to give her consent and he would have most of the children of the prostitutes at his school. He did not want to waste another moment. We drove to Satara, and to the house of the Madam 'of the field'. On the way we discussed the double dilemma created by his breakthrough: the children's mothers were paying the school fees out of their sex-work; and now, by looking after the children, the mothers were available to do more sex-work. Randive's predicament with the prostitutes made me think of Major Barbara Undershaft, George Bernard Shaw's compromised heroine in his controversial play of 1907, 'Major Barbara', who resigns after the Salvation Army accept a donation from her father, the arms manufacturer. The idealistic heroine is prepared to stop ministering to the poor, rather than accept dirty money. Randive didn't know the play, but he recognised the compromise – 'the tempering of idealism by reality.' Did Randive feel compromised at having to receive payment from prostitutes? Randive said that the prostitutes were the abused party in this situation. And he could not wait for the problem of prostitution to go away before helping their children. He would like to create – and had tried – alternative work for the women, but these schemes could not match the money they earned selling their bodies. It took a lot of trust, even courage, for a young woman to walk away from work that gave them a measure of security. Building that trust took time. And it took hope. Randive believed that by having their children at his school the sex-workers would be one-remove from seeing a better way and finding hope, the elusive but essential ingredient needed for change. HIV/AIDS had actually opened a door for Randive. Some women – discovering their status – had abandoned the work. I had met one of them, Sunita, a formidable woman who had been instrumental in helping Randive get to know the Madams of Satara. After discovering her status, Sunita had started a jewellery business and now made enough to live and support her own child. She was only one person; but in the alternative economy of Randive's work one changed lifestyle represented the ultimate success.

The Madam of the field's house was in the better part of town. It was tidily furnished, thoughtfully decorated and had all the home comforts, including armchairs and a big television upon which her teenage sons were playing Play Station. A motorbike was parked in the kitchen. Out the back, in the yard, there were four rooms where her girls slept. The sons of the Madam (how I wanted to hear their stories) left the room and we gathered in a circle on the floor: the Madam, looking smart in a white sari flecked with gold, and four of her girls. Another girl stood in the alcove; she had long, shiny, well-groomed hair and wore a smart trouser suit. The Madam said to Randive that this was the girl who had run away from her husband and was seeking shelter. Randive was greatly excited. He asked her to join us. He then asked her what she intended to do. The Madam repeated her claim that she did not want this girl to do any sex-work; but the girl had said she would rather do sex-work than go back to her husband. Randive said that he would help her find a place to stay if she promised not to do that. The Madam repeated her position and she and Randive agreed to help this girl to avoid ending up in the sex business. There was something powerful about this transaction: the Madam, caught in a delicate balance between exploiting girls and pastoring them, did not want this girl to end up like her and the other women in the room. It was a tacit acknowledgment that there was a better life; and that this life they had chosen was a last resort.

'So, Benjamin,' I said. 'It has been a good week. You have talked to about three hundred people about HIV/AIDS; you have rescued a girl from prostitution, and you have persuaded the Madams – including the Madam of the Sex Field – to pay for the children of the sex-workers to go to your school.'

He laughed. 'I have been working on this problem for four long years,' he said, 'And in one day this happens. If I take these children, maybe 50% of their mothers will change.'

'Can people really change, Major?'

'People are longing for something better but no one is there to show the way.'

'You're there. Ratnamala. Pria. Timothy. Pravin. All the team.'

Randive took off his glasses and wiped his eyes as we drove away from the Madam's house. I had not really noticed it until now, but Randive was a handsome man and when he smiled it was hard not to smile with him.

'I would like to buy presents for your family. Something from India,' he said.

'You don't have to, Major.'

'Yes. It is my pleasure.'

The vehicle careened along, weaving through the late-afternoon traffic in the city. Satara did not improve in the dusk light; it was intrinsically ugly; as is sometimes said in the guide books of indistinct places you pass through on the way to somewhere of touristic value, Satara had no redeeming features. Unless you count Major Randive and his like.

'Would you like to be posted somewhere more beautiful than here, Major? Do you have a favourite place, a dream place you would like to go to?'

'I have been 25 years in Salvation Army. I have been here four years. I don't have a favourite place because God has called me to serve. Good place, bad place.'

'And how do you keep going? Keep your spirits up?'

'The Salvation Army is my motivation. My wife is my back up. My daughter is my personal assistant. God gives me energy.'

I made a tape about Randive for the World Service, hoping to capture something of the man's quiet heroism and thinking how much more he deserved than five minutes radio time from me. But it isn't in the Salvation Army's nature to single out soldiers for special honours; Randive's kind of uncomplaining servant-hood is in the job description. There were other saints doing unsung work, no less difficult than him, all over the world. He was emblematic of this work, but still only one player in a cast of thousands who live out hidden subplots of quiet drama, trying to subvert the seemingly inevitable destructive course of the main story through small acts of kindness. But I couldn't fully stop myself from singling him out. He was an inspiration and the young men in Kithituni had spoken of how it was the example of others – Rebecca, Ian, Mark – that had inspired them to do the work. Maybe when you can create enough Randives the small stories become the Big Story.

The Needle and the Damage Done

The HIV virus only has to latch on to the coat-tails of mankind's addictions for it to be carried to new places where it can thrive. An unhappy meeting of limited economic and social opportunity and a proximity to drug trafficking had made Mizoram one of these places. This north-eastern Indian state squats between Bangladesh in the west and Myanmar (formerly Burma) in the east, adjacent to what is cynically and sentimentally called The Golden Triangle, one of Asia's two main illicit opium-producing areas. Mizoram is an easy conduit for the trafficking of heroin into India and hits from this activity had bruised the minds and bodies of many who inhabit this quiet, gently mountainous country.

In Aizawl, the principal town of Mizoram, a man called John rolled up his trousers and showed us the bruised fruit of his former addiction. For several years he had injected himself with a combination of prescription drugs: Proxyvon (or Spas), a synthetic opoid painkiller, and the sedative Nitrazepam. He'd tried other things, including Polyfiller (his lower legs actually looked like the damp walls of an old house that had been filled in and papered over too many times and it was uncomfortable watching him touch the brittle, puce contusions in case they cracked in).

'See,' he said, opening his hands, palms up. His hands displayed the addict's genius for finding space for injecting where there should be none.

'These are my scars.'

My children looked at John's hands and feet and were rightly amazed that someone would do this to themselves in the pursuit of pleasure.

'Yuck.'

John laughed and nodded in agreement.

My children were getting a simple and effective lesson in the dangers of taking drugs.

John's story was almost archetypal for young men here: unemployed but trying to scrape a living, he'd got a job carrying heroin for a dealer across the border in Myanmar. One day he tried heroin (after all, it was one of the 'perks' of the job). Addiction swooped and he was soon incapable of couriering. He lost his job and the easy access to his drug of choice so he moved on to cheaper, more accessible drugs. Then, six years ago, he discovered that he was HIV positive. HIV infection was only detected in Mizoram in 1990 and at that time, 90% of injecting drug-users were sharing needles and syringes without adequate cleaning.

Maia, John's wife, was sitting with a young baby in a sheet for a sling, on the bed next to her husband. She was also infected, although their child was not. Most drug-users in Mizoram were male. Women only made up 10% of drug-users here but they were greatly affected as they bore the burden of looking after family members who were addicted. Maia had been with John when he became an addict and she had stuck with him right through his addiction. But towards the end it became impossible and she sought help through the Salvation Army.

'CHAN* saved my life,' John said. He nodded at Jimmy and George, who were volunteers with the Salvation Army's community network, and our accompaniment for our time in Mizoram. From the window of John's house, we could see the city of Aizawl – at least a part of it. Concrete buildings clung to steep slopes all the way down in to the valley. The city was a collection of peaks and each peak was concrete clad. The vista

---

* CHAN – Community Health Action Network.

fooled you for a moment: it created the impression that Aizawl was a beautiful town and if you half closed your eyes and didn't focus on individual buildings, it almost was. But Aizawl was a haphazard, characterless place, choked with the pollution of diesel-burning traffic. A town with no real centre, like the state of Mizoram, it wasn't sure who or what it was. It was Indian, but the people looked more Chinese; it was mountainous but the air was not fresh; we were hemmed in by the great religions of the world, but 80% of the population went to church.

The pattern of drug use in Mizoram had changed in the last thirty years. It started when young people tried smoking heroin in the 1970s and this evolved into heroin injecting in the 1980s. The highly addictive drug was a double disaster: it demanded more of the same, quickly, and it was expensive; and the expense of the drug saw people turn to other, cheaper drugs and then prostitution in order to pay for the habit. Meanwhile HIV had all the conditions it needed to flourish: a growing community of drugs users who shared needles and financed its addiction through becoming part of the sex-trade. By the 1990s a concentrated epidemic among these users had become a generalised epidemic, crossing over into the lives of non-drug-users who were related to addicts. John's wife was an example of this.

The government had been active in responding: the Ministry for Social Justice provided grants – in aid to about 375 NGOs for drug-addiction schemes, of which 46 NGOs functioned exclusively in the north-eastern states. And Mizoram was full of Self-Help Groups (SHGs – there will always be an acronym). But the philosophies weren't always joined up.

The government itself had recently tried a more blunt interventionist approach in the form of a 'boot camp' (their own name) for users and pushers, as well as sex-workers.

Jimmy and George took us to see it, knowing full well that it would be a good advertisement for 'how not to deal with the problem'. And so it was. The boot camp was a dismal, enervating place, like an under-funded boarding school for dropouts on a three-month detention. It was a shallow response and the statistics bore this out. Most of the young people I talked to there did not expect to be cured of their addictions.

Jimmy and George took me to see the General Secretary of the Positive Network – a support group, backed by the Salvation Army, that did what it said on the tin: it connected people with HIV in the community and encouraged them to support each other.

The office of the Positive Network was a room, partitioned at one end to provide a private counselling space, with four chairs and a desk. Some AIDS awareness posters on the peeling walls brightened the spartan décor. The General Secretary was not as frightening or as senior as his title suggested. Mongia was a young man in his twenties, an ex-heroin addict and HIV positive; he was serious, structured and articulate about his role.

'We have a lot of visions, dreams for the HIV people in Aizawl. One. To make sure that in the next ten years that HIV will not be shameful – that they will not be outcast. That the people can expose themselves freely. Stigmatisation is still very high. Especially in the villages. Many don't have the courage to go back to the villages. Two. More than 80% of HIV people live below the poverty line. And there are many deaths through lack of medication. We want to make sure they get the proper medication, support and counselling. And three. We want to reach out to all the HIV positive people who are still on drugs, help them maintain a clean life, a sober life and have a new life in Christ which is helpful for them and the nation.'

Mongia said this last sentence without any guile or equivocation. The connection between transformation and faith was a given for him. I could have dismissed it as the expected, handed down belief of a young man growing up in a Christian state; but for

Mongia it was personal.

'Does faith really make a difference?' I asked him.

'I believe the ones who have faith will live healthier and longer. I have not only seen it, I have experienced it myself. There was nothing that could get me off the drugs – not even my parents who loved me the most. Faith in Jesus helped me. The life in Christ really changes a person. Counselling is not enough. People don't want to come into the network…they want something more. Those who have the life in Christ, who come off the streets, are happier and healthier. They don't have so much sadness and sickness and pain in the mind and body.'

'So how do you introduce addicts to Jesus?'

'We have to meet people where they are. Full acceptance of a person's beliefs is necessary to build a rapport and trust. Most people who come don't really have any faith. But they are full of despair. And fear. And they are desperate. Working in the field is not easy. It is more than a day-to-day job. It takes a lifetime. At the same time the Holy Spirit can do things beyond what we can do, so we are at peace doing this job.'

Faith and hope. When the programme was stripped down to its essentials these were the two vital ingredients in this HIV/AIDS response. It was these things that gave it stickability; as Mongia put it, 'We are at peace with doing this job – despite it being hard and slow and sometimes hard to see change.' Faith gave the programme a sustainability it might otherwise not have had.

But Mizoram had many NGOs offering programmes and support for people with HIV/AIDS. How did they see the approach of the faith-based Churches? I thought I'd start with the biggest so I went to interview Lelupui Silu who worked for the UN office of Drugs and Crime in Aizawl.

I put it to her. 'There are lots of people doing good work but are they doing it together?'

'Most NGOs here are dealing with drugs and HIV. They started independently but over the last four or five years they've started networking. For example they support each other with resources, from dressing, to food, to shelter.'

'And what is your view of the Salvation Army approach?'

'The Salvation Army initiated a response before anyone else – even the government. The biggest plus point that they have is being in the community. This is so important, whatever the health or social issue. The Salvation Army are already there, alongside them. That is where I see the light. They actually connect a lot of NGOs to the community that we couldn't otherwise reach. For any programme to be sustained, it needs ownership. Since the Salvation Army is in the community, the programme will go on whether the funds come or not.'

'But do all these NGOs agree about how to tackle the problem? Do they love each other?'

'Sometimes yes. Sometimes no. There is a big gulf between theory and practice. For example it was thought reaching clients was easy but this is the most time consuming part. Connecting. Being present. And it's expensive. Sex-workers are mobile and fragile, therefore hard to follow. Our sex-workers are not brothel based; they operate on their own which is much harder to reach them. And meeting once is not enough. Unless you are with these people, alongside them, then you cannot know what they really face. This is the challenge for all NGOs. How to be alongside the people.'

A month later, when we had returned to Kithituni, we would meet a friend of April Foster's – Pierre Robert – who worked for UNESCO. Pierre had worked in Mali on a series of HIV/AIDS initiatives there and had seen all kinds of different responses to the problem. He was an atheist – 'Sometimes I'm an agnostic' – but when I asked him about a faith-based approach to the problem he said:

'The "faith guys" take a long view. They have an eternal perspective, I guess, that keeps them going. It usually means their motivation comes from a deeper place – it's not about career, or feeling better about themselves, or meeting a particular target. It's like they're operating to a bigger plan. It's not about them. To help the people you have to be willing to give things up and not care about yourself. Not everyone can do that. People with faith seem to be better equipped in this respect. The faith guys don't have to worry about looking good to the world.'

After Mizoram, we flew back to Kenya via the great Indian delta city of Calcutta, a place synonymous with poverty and charity. We stayed in the heart of the city, near the Salvation Army guest-house and its brazen sign advertising 'Mass Feeding of the Poor Every Sunday.' We saw the tatty tigers, flea-bitten and skinny, in the appalling Calcutta Zoo; we treated ourselves to silk bedspreads from the bazaar and a full-blown five-course meal. We then completed the 'Calcutta tourist trail' with a visit to see the Sisters of Mercy Convent and the statue of its most famous resident.

We went and stood before the statue of Mother Teresa. For many people the bar for goodness doesn't get any higher than this. Here was the acme of saintliness. But I couldn't work out if her repute was inspiring or intimidating; did her example call us to go and be saints or did her canonisation send out the message that doing good things was for super saints – not for people like you and me. I'd like to have met her, or seen her in action, but her statue and the little bits of memorabilia left me cold. Only her simple, stripped-down bedroom – the room where she'd slept all those years – seemed to tell us something about the woman. But I'm not sure goodness is something to enshrine or put in a display case. As Pierre Robert said: 'the faith guys don't have to worry about looking good to the world.'

'Just Like In That Movie'

From India we returned to Africa and continued on into the more deeply affected regions of the pandemic. After a brief fuel stop and re-hydration, in what had effectively become our base camp in Kithituni, Kenya, we set off again on a road that would take us to the Kibera – Nairobi's vast slum – and then on to Rwanda and Uganda, where the pandemic had already done its worst.

In the Sarit Centre, one of Nairobi's main shopping malls, a young man was selling counterfeit DVDs, some with as many as ten movies on one disc.

'Here,' he said, holding up a disc with a sleeve depicting the English actor, Ralph Fiennes looking handsome and concerned. 'They make this here in Kibera. I live in Kibera, just like in that movie.'

The man said he wanted to go to college but he didn't have the funds so, to make a living, he sold movies to people who were rich enough to have their own DVD players. That meant coming to the Sarit Centre, where Nairobi's affluent citizens came to shop. On a good day he could make a thousand shillings (£20) which made him rich compared to the average Kenyan who tried to live on two or three thousand shillings per month. As part of his sales patter he mentioned that one of his two children had died last year from pneumonia, the result of AIDS.

Like most of the hawkers in the mall, the man worked itinerantly by day and returned, at sundown, to the largest slum in Africa – the Kibera – a shanty-town no more than a twenty-minute vulture glide from the reassuring consumerism of the mall. I declined his offer, not because I didn't want to buy his illegal merchandise but because we had just seen that movie on DVD – *The Constant Gardener* – only two days before. Based on the novel by John le Carré, it tells the story of a diplomat (played by Fiennes) who tries to piece together the reasons for his wife's murder and in the process unveils a conspiracy involving a pharmaceutical company that used the Kibera as a test ground for its new tuberculosis and HIV/AIDS drugs. *The Constant Gardener* was praised for its gritty realism and for being shot on location in Kenya. It was directed by Fernando Meirelles, who had made *City Of God*, a film set in the slums of Rio. I was curious to see if our own impending visit to the Kibera would show the movie to be as realistic as the critics were saying.

The idea that drug companies test their products on unsuspecting Africans is another myth to add to a building mythology of HIV/AIDS conspiracy theories. Many of these concern the origins of the disease itself. Some say AIDS started in the 'dark continent', then spread to Haiti, then to the United States and to Europe, another infestation from the so-called Third World (surely a descriptor ripe for replacement seeing as the conditions that define 'Third World' are found where most of the world lives). In these theories, Africa is seen as the cradle of AIDS and with this come a set of stereotypes about a primitive past, and transmission from animals' sexual license. A counter myth (which has some serious minded advocates) says that the virus was sent to Africa from the United States, an act of bacterial warfare to decrease the African birth rate. This story has the virus created in a CIA-Army laboratory, sent to Africa, and then brought back to the United States by American homosexual missionaries returning from Africa. In October 1985 a Soviet weekly published an article alleging that the AIDS virus had been engineered by the US government. A year later the UK newspaper the *Sunday Express* ran a story that claimed 'Killer AIDS Virus was Artificially Created by American Scientists.' This story was repeated in papers all over the world. The trouble with *The Constant Gardener* was that it did what these other myths did: it focused our attention on the wrong thing: evil pharmaceutical companies conspiring, Western governments exploiting, corrupt African governments failing to act; ideas that leave us none the wiser, and perhaps even less sympathetic to the issue. Big picture issues that make for movies but don't account for the little acts.

Meanwhile, the reality is, of course, more prosaic: as we leave the mall a man carrying a bag of medicine and a prescription stops us and says he is HIV positive and needs three hundred shillings (£4) to get one last bottle of medicine. If someone gives him the change he needs, he gets the drugs and lives. Such are the dull, unfilmed scenes that make up the unfolding story of AIDS.

It was morning as we drove towards the slum that some say is 'the biggest in Africa'. We moved against a human tide: stadium sized crowds loping along the sides of Nairobi's roads. Striding in clusters of twos and threes the people were pouring out of the Kibera in search of casual labour, hoping to pick up work with one of the construction companies or perhaps some ancillary job in a hotel or a restaurant.

We were with Douglas Jigali, a PSS (psycho–social–support) worker with the Salvation Army who worked mainly with the children who had lost a parent or parents to HIV/AIDS. Douglas was in his late twenties and had lived in the Kibera for eight years. I was hoping he could help me clarify this issue of how many people lived in the slum. I had been told that the Kibera housed a quarter of Nairobi's population and yet most people I asked said it contained a million, even 1.5 million. My guidebook said the population of Nairobi was 2.1 million but didn't mention the Kibera at all. It simply said: 'Nairobi has scenes of shocking poverty, so if you are worried stay in one of the affluent suburbs rather than the downtown dives.' It then directed people to the country's wildlife.

'The number is always about one million.' Douglas said. 'Even though people are always coming and going, the numbers are the same. There is never an empty house in the Kibera. When somebody leaves, it's immediately filled.'

Douglas was married and had a six-month-old baby. He lived, as we were about to see, in a cupboard-sized room on the Salvation Army compound at the far edge of the slum. When he talked about the Kibera, he talked about it with affection.

'I like the place. The Kibera is a slum but living is cheap. Less than a dollar a day gets you meals. Sanitation is the main problem. But life is good compared to some places. It is the cheapest place to stay. It means people can come to the city and afford to look for work. They come to look for a job. The majority come here because they know someone – a friend or a family member – who is here. You need a relative.'

'And what work will they find – all these people here we are passing on the streets?'

'Nearly all these people are casuals. They end up wandering for work. Usually ladies wash up. Men become hard labourers. But at least they don't need much money to survive in the slum.'

Our vehicle passed a sign saying 'Nairobi City Council' and an arrow pointing to Kibera Primary School. The buildings suddenly changed. The colours changed. The atmosphere changed: from the wannabe internationalist concrete corporate of Nairobi Central to single storey mud and corrugated iron shack; from mildly threatening and bland to anarchically communal and loud.

'We are entering the Kibera now,' Douglas said.

He pointed to a patch of open land and said that this was where former Kenyan president Daniel Arap Moi had been born. Apparently the government owned this land on which the Kibera had grown and they wanted it back.

'Maybe they should swap,' I joked. 'Come and live here. Let the people camp on the presidential grass – like the protesting Masai and their cattle.'

Douglas took me literally. 'No. The government would not want to give up their nice places for this.'

A heap of refuse, twice the height of a man, sat uncollected at the side of the road. The road itself was no longer tarmac but a compressed dust mud road like that in the village back in Kithituni. People criss-crossed the roads and we slowed to a walking pace as we were now entering a place where roads were for people not cars. We passed another pile of uncollected waste, stacked to the height of the one storey shacks which again were more like the market stalls back in the country towns. The shops looked colourful and we caught snatches of music as we passed them.

'This is the better part of the Kibera here. The buildings get worse as you go down the slope into the valley.'

Still it was hard to get a sense of scale. Or numbers.

Signage decorated the shack fronts and cluttered the streets. Signs were the dominant form of expression in the Kibera and they were funny: consciously ironic of the credibility gap between what was being offered and the context of their surroundings, a kind of defiant, inverted civic pride. There were the commercial stalls: Karibu (meaning 'welcome' in Swahili) Hotel; Jamina Tailoring; Mama Sisters Salon (hundreds of hair salons); The Moscow Butchery; Simba Artists; His Mercy's Salon. All of them seemed to be doing a good trade. Then there were the churches – all denominations were here. The one with the biggest sign being the Samaritan's Ark Church. Then the NGOs, the internationally renowned and the homemade, (the Kibera was an opportunity for many to raise funds). There was even a Constant Gardener Trust here. During filming the cast and crew decided to set up an organisation that, initially, would help the communities they had met and worked with during the shoot. Their aim: 'to help improve basic sanitation and education for those that are most in need of our help.' They said that they were a small organisation, hoping to achieve big things and a new ethos of responsible filmmaking along the way. To achieve this they believed that the best and most lasting change comes through careful thought and collaboration with the people we are trying to help. We had not seen this many NGOs gathered in one place, nor would we again see its like. I ventured to Douglas that all this support must have made a difference. 'Yes, but most NGOs work independently. There is minimal networking. I would like to see more networking. There are some people (especially those with HIV) you find attached to several NGOs while others are not attached to even one. Some benefit more than others. And it is usually the neediest who are not good at getting help.' There it was again: a lack of joined up thinking. Plenty of good will and support; but too many agendas to push and few prepared to surrender their advantage (or their funding).

Other agencies left signs announcing their contribution to the Kibera. The most flagrantly jarring was painted on a wall next to a row of eight green toilets that had been donated by UNICEF (which also had a discreet sign). In big, fresh colours it said 'We're Wash Compliant – We Perform Well.' It was hard to tell who the 'we' were and you had to wonder how bad things would be if they hadn't been performing well. There is no running water in the Kibera and refuse is collected once a month, sometimes once every two months. Whoever the 'wash compliant guys' were they must have been operating in some other place of their own imagining. There is an average of one pit latrine for every five hundred people in the slum. Drinking water is there but it is pumped through brittle and easily broken plastic pipes that run alongside the sewage trenches that carry the waste to the river at the base of the valley.

'So where do people go to the toilet?'

Douglas explained. 'In Kibera, we have flying toilets. The

people do it in the plastic shopping bags and then throw the bag over their fence or wall. If you don't like your neighbour you know what you can do.'

The vehicle pulled off the mud track, through a set of gates, and we entered a Salvation Army compound that consisted of a church building, a school, a community centre, a garden and a house. The stink of un-drained human excrement and uncollected waste hit us once we got out of the vehicle. The site was about one hundred metres by eighty metres; it was an island or, as Douglas said, 'an oasis' in a desert devoid of natural beauty. The compound even had flowers and trees, planted so people would get some sense of respite when they came here. If it wasn't for the smell, you wouldn't have guessed where you were.

The compound had gates but it wasn't a gated community, protecting its own and failing to engage with what lay outside the gates (like the residences of the rich communities in Nairobi and Johannesburg). The compound and its facilities were available to many different groups to use. HIV/AIDS awareness meetings regularly took place in the community centre.

Crucially, the Salvation Army didn't just have an office here, they lived here. Captain N'Donke and his wife, Grace, had come here from western Kenya and had been here now for two years. We were invited into their quarters which were clean and uniform and had that kitsch Victoriana décor we would encounter in officers' houses from Kigali to Calcutta: a kind of tea and doily, lace curtain fastidiousness that in the Kibera seemed like a radical statement of victory for cleanliness and order over filth and chaos. Grace took crockery from a glass cabinet that had the Salvation Army logo – 'Blood and Fire' – carved into the wood. She served us tea and biscuits and her husband, a serious, intelligent man economically summarised for me the essential issue faced by the people of the Kibera.

Poverty.

'There are many things people cannot accomplish because of

poverty. They don't get enough food. They can't afford treatment – many people die simply because they don't get treatment. When people need medicine, most rely on free medical centres. Government. Hospitals don't have adequate facilities. People get drugs sometimes but not with prescription. So they get the wrong medicine.'

I asked the Captain if he had seen the movie *The Constant Gardener*. The Captain said he had not seen the movie although he had heard of it because tourists had come to the slum because of it. For the Captain it came down to a lack of political will. A lack of joined up thinking. It wasn't about drug companies using the poor as guinea pigs, it was about drug companies – and governments – not making drugs affordable to the poor. Only a few days before our visit we had been sick with stomach bugs since our return from India; because we were rich and connected enough we had gone to the smart and efficient Nairobi outpatient clinic and been prescribed drugs (for typhoid) that had cost us £64 – an impossible amount of money for someone living here.

Douglas was worried about the rain: he pointed to the grey clouds gathering outside. Since our return from India the weather had turned and it had started to rain the way it should and needed to; but in the slum this was no cause for celebration. Unlike most parts of Kenya, rain in the Kibera is not welcomed or prayed or danced over. When it rains the water turns the sloping roads into slopping rivers and the back and side alleys into stinking streams, all the detritus flowing down into the valley below us and forming a River of Shit that flows on down to Nairobi Dam where people play and wash, bath and clean their clothes. This is a visible iniquity that should be remedied and isn't. The captain said that some day there could be a serious outbreak of typhoid or cholera here.

We went first to the school on the compound. The school's outside corrugated iron wall was bright turquoise and someone had painted four *Richard Scarry* animals on it. My very first book was *Richard Scarry's Big Schoolbook*. How Lowly the Worm would have loved the mud and decay of this place. Inside the schoolroom a class of about thirty children aged between three and maybe nine, stood to attention. The teacher – an immaculately dressed woman – asked them to say hello. It was the first class of children I had seen where the pupils were not in a specific uniform. Smartly dressed African school children (no matter the poverty of their circumstances) were a constant motif on this journey. I understood the reasons for uniform – the dignity, the collective purpose, the fairness – but it sometimes seemed ridiculous to think of parents straining to get the money together for uniforms when there were schools without books. Here, uniform was out of the question. Many of these children were orphans, or had lost one parent to HIV/AIDS. But the children were as bright and cheerful as any we had met. How children manage to be like this, no matter where they are, is a mystery worthy of study in itself.

The children all stood and began to recite rhymes in English. First they sang 'The Rain In Spain', then 'Rain, Rain Go Away'. How odd to listen to these African children singing, without irony, rhymes about a subject that for us is conversation and for them a matter of life and death.

Before continuing with our walk through the Kibera, Douglas told me to climb the compound fence and take a look: I would be able to see much of the slum from this vantage point. I stepped upon the wall and shinnied up the wooden fence to see. Immediately I realised that I had already seen this view – in the movie. The two essential differences between that view and this were the tone and the smell. In the film – even a film striving for authentic grit – the sprawling shanty town had a golden hue and it almost glowed; without filters it looked a dull rust brown. But the real difference was something the thing a film couldn't capture. The movie had caught the colour and something of the vibrancy of the slum, but it couldn't capture the smell, and without the smell you only

121

get half the picture; without the smell you might be fooled into thinking this was a tolerable place to live.

The name Kibera is a Nubian word for 'forest'. The original settlers were Sudanese soldiers sent to build the railway after returning from fighting in the First World War for the British. They made their homes in the railway sidings. I presume there were trees here once. Now it is a forest of wires and plastic sheeting and tin in a valley (more gulley) of single storey shacks and a network of back alleys spreading as far as I could see. I was looking out over most of the Kibera's nine official villages: Kianda, Soweto, Gatwekera, Kisumu Ndogo, Lindi, Laini Saba, Siranga/Undugu, Makina and Mashimoni. I was told that the average home in the Kibera was three metres by three metres with an average of five people per dwelling, but I found it hard to believe I was looking at the largest 'informal' settlement in Africa. It didn't seem a big enough space to contain a million people.

Just beneath my nose, a flying toilet's throw from the compound, I could see a mother, with her two children, washing clothes and hanging them on a line tied between a wooden fence and a wall seemingly constructed from plastic sheets. The clothes on the line and on her children were miraculously clean – cleaner than my own children's clothes – and they smiled at me, amused that I would want to take a picture of such a thing.

Walking through the Kibera was like walking through a city sprouting up from a garbage dump. The garbage lay everywhere, in great stinking heaps, right outside fruit stalls and hair salons. The mud and the rain and the slant of the road meant little rivulets of detritus ran randomly towards the valley floor. As we walked I became conscious of my feet, more particularly my children's feet. My daughter was wearing open-toed sandals and her legs were bare. We had been surrounded and almost permanently accompanied by shoeless children for weeks but I couldn't stop looking at her feet and began to fuss at her, telling her to be careful where she trod. My son pulled up his Manchester United shirt over his nose to muffle the stink.

Around the first corner we came across a man stirring what looked like scummy water in an oil barrel. He was making maize beer. Sitting on child-sized chairs beneath the overhang of his roof, six men sat imbibing this stuff. They all seemed inebriated, their eyes big and sleepy and bloodshot. This kind of beer is easily contaminated with bad water, or mixed with the wrong proportions of alcohol or a toxic wood – as in the tragic case of the Machakos disaster in June 2005, when 174 people were hospitalised and 49 people died after drinking a homemade brew that contained methanol.

Inebriated men in front of shacks. This image was recurring and would continue to recur. Were these men being sociable or were they escaping something? They asked us to join them for a brew but we were with a teetotal organisation and our stomachs were still struggling from bugs picked up in India. Despite this there was not any aggression or threat in this scene. In Nairobi Central I had felt far more afraid; there was a real sense of danger there; here it was different. In the city people were wary and walked faster, here people seemed to want to talk. The Kibera was less a city, more a shambling village that had got completely out of hand.

Around the next corner I saw two children hop-scotching across a trench carrying away brown water.

Then the street straightened out and we could see the Kibera spreading before us. More garbage and more shop fronts. Every dwelling seemed to double as some kind of shop. We stopped at a hair salon. It was run by Anna, a woman in her thirties. I asked her how many heads per day she serviced. She said between five and ten but that she needed about a hundred to make ends meet. She employed three people. She was also HIV positive and had discovered her status four years before. She said she was doing okay, considering, but her children were not at school and the

ARVs were expensive. She talked to anyone about AIDS, warning them of the dangers. 'AIDS is a big problem in Kibera.' (I tried to get accurate statistics about the prevalence rates in the Kibera and got a range from one in five to one in three adults being HIV positive. Either way much higher than the national Kenyan average of 7%.)

Across the street, opposite the salon, big music and laughter came from the pool hall that was the headquarters of 'Visionary Youth', a self-help group that was started here in response to the HIV/AIDS crisis. It had only been going for a year but it had two hundred members – all young men. William, the 'club secretary', was at the table leaning on his cue, hat flipped back. He looked high, maybe drunk, but he was keen to advocate the seriousness and sobriety of this group, which used pool as the hook and magnet.

'We play tournament in Kisumu. We are good. We go to America. Anywhere. As long as it's a foreign country.'

'Do you drink beer?'

'No home brew here. That is evil,' he said.

'You talk about HIV? Safe sex.'

'Yes. Men don't always talk. Women better. So pool helps. We preach safe sex.'

The men all laughed at their leader. Some of them invited us to join them and play a game.

Entering Kibera I had a series of reactions from the indignant: 'How on earth can people live like this?' to the amazed: 'Look how alive this place is.' For a moment I almost felt envy at the anarchic connectedness of the community and the fact that the people looked happier here than back in the capital's smart coffee bars. Did I imagine this or are the people who live here more friendly, more communicative, more connected than those of us living in astonishing luxury? And if it is the case is it because a lack of stuff levels out the competitive, covetous inclinations that material wealth can induce? Or were these the luxurious musings of a man who strolls through the abject, stinking city in the sure and certain knowledge of having a hot, clean bath at the end of it, in which he might wash off the grime and the muck from his daughter's feet?

We walked on through the slum for another half hour and still we couldn't see its end. We stepped over the train tracks, the original line where the settlement started here years before: a line that runs all the way east, past Makindu and Kithituni and Sultan Hamud and on to the sea port of Mombasa, built to ferry goods out of Africa and back to Britain. We had walked for 25 minutes and still we could see shacks everywhere. As we stepped along the tracks, we could sense the movement of people heading off the streets and into their three-by-threes.

'We must get back soon.' Douglas said. It was starting to rain.

As we walked back to the compound we were followed by a man who looked drunk. He asked us who we were and what we were doing and then began to tell us his life-story which with every step we took made us less sympathetic towards him. He had been a student but had run out of funds because he had got sick. He also had fathered a child but the mother had left him for another man. That was when he started drinking. His drinking led him to flunk college and use all his money. And then he had discovered that he was HIV positive.

This last detail was thrown in with a dramatic flourish, the *coup de grâce* that would surely hook this Westerner into giving up funds. But I was not listening; I was taking my cue from the captain who said he had heard this man's story before and it always changed in every detail except for that last part: the request for money. It was a familiar story and one full of half-truth and self-pity. Finding no succour from me the man turned to my son, walking a few yards behind me, gingerly avoiding the muck on the road. He struck up a conversation but I didn't like it and motioned to Gabriel to join me. Then my daughter, who had some Kenyan shillings, spontaneously offered to give the man her money. He was going to take it when I stopped her, angry at him for taking advantage of a six-year-old.

'No!' I said.

The man finally gave up on us and walked off, talking quite loudly to himself.

'What is wrong with that man?' My daughter asked me.

'He's…' but I couldn't think what to say.

'Why couldn't I give him the money?' she persisted.

'Because money isn't what he needs,' I said.

Agnes didn't look convinced. I wasn't either. I thought about using the 'it's better to teach a man to fish than give a man a fish' line; but I thought better of it. Agnes would probably have said something like: 'Yeah, but what's he going to eat until he knows how to fish properly?' Or worse: 'Why don't you teach him to fish?'

As we walked deeper into the community, over mountains of ordure, you could see, behind the smiles, that there was a daily battle going on that no amount of NGOs providing toilets could alleviate. The indignation rose. Surely a society that has the wit and the will to put a cup of latte on a table but one mile from here can find a way to clear the garbage that kills people every day; where is the connection between the deals done by statesmen and this struggle for daily living? When are we going to measure the greatness of nations by the way they treat their poorest instead of by the kilowatts of power they generate? A slum says many things. The danger for us is that if we don't like what we hear we disconnect: we make sure the presidential plane avoids the slum side of the city, we fail to mention them in our books; we do our bit, then walk away and wash the shit from our feet. Meanwhile people like Douglas and the Captain and his wife – people who can see and smell as well as the rest of us – choose to stay. Maybe it's easier for them to do this when they believe in a God who was born in a pigsty and died on a hill of decaying garbage.

Où Est Le Docteur?

If you were dropped into Rwanda with no knowledge of its recent history; dropped, say, into a village nestling into one of the country's thousand hills, the thing you'd most likely notice first is the landscape: how lush, how green, how panoramic. You might see the people, teeming upon the steep terraces, tilling the soil or working in luminous fields of tea, silver eucalyptus and banana. From this you might deduce that you'd stepped into some pastoral idyll, where the land and its people were fruitful and content and had been so for centuries. You'd probably think the landscape so beautiful that you'd wonder if this really was the place where one of the world's worst atrocities had happened just twelve years before.

You arrive in Rwanda with such a pornography of bad imagery that the shock of the beauty of the landscape really catches you out. In the first few days of our visit – and particularly once we got out of the city – we found ourselves continually telling people we met how beautiful their country was.

'*Quel beau pays. Votre pays. Le pays: c'est très beau,*' we enthused.

This wasn't to flatter them. It was a statement of fact and a fact exaggerated because we hadn't expected it. Except for Johnnie Boy, from Kithituni, who had never been anywhere other than Kenya until he came here to see the AIDS response work, no one had told us that Rwanda was beautiful. It wasn't the thing to mention.

Our comments weren't received with looks of knowing pride by the people, more with looks of surprise, as if this self-evident truth had not occurred to them.

'*Tu crois? Peut-être.*'

As the days went by we stopped our complimenting. Rwandans probably knew they lived in a beautiful country, but they had forgotten the fact, or chosen to forget; how can you praise the landscape when it had been the silent stage upon which such appalling things have happened?

Just as in India and Mizoram and Kenya – everywhere we went – AIDS amplified a country's existing ills and weaknesses; in Rwanda it had proved as merciless as the genocidaires who had decimated the population. Buried in that dead decimal lay other awful superlatives: 200,000 women raped. 100,000 people needing HIV treatment; 260,000 orphans; 65,000 of them HIV positive.

I tried to explain to my children what genocide was in general and what the Rwandan genocide was in particular; a task I found slightly more awkward than explaining prostitution. Again, I had to try and work out what detail to include and what to censor. I tried to explain how one group of people – the Hutu – had killed another group – the Tutsi. I gave them the key number – one million people killed in one hundred days (the Rwandan genocide was a proper decimation: the killing of every tenth person in a population) – but I didn't mention that it had been done with machetes (later, when they visited the genocide museum in Kigali, they would see how it had been done and be disgusted).

Then my son asked me why.

How to explain – to a child or even an adult – the most efficient mass killing since the atomic bombings of Hiroshima and Nagasaki? I had come well-armed with explanation. I had read the books – *We Wish To Inform You That Tomorrow We Will Be Killed With Our Families* by Philip Gourevitch being among the best of them; I had seen the movie *Hotel Rwanda*; I had read the news articles;

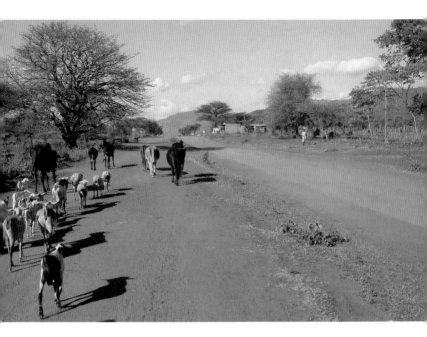

The red road to Kithituni, Kenya

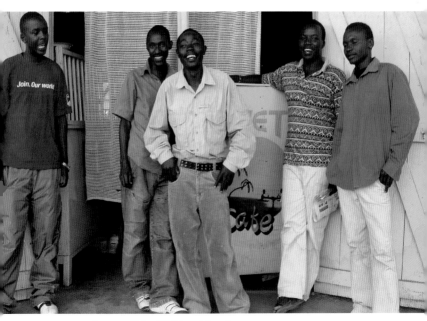

Some of the Kithituni local response team:
Johnnie Boy, Mark, Georgie-Porgie, Onesmus and Joseph

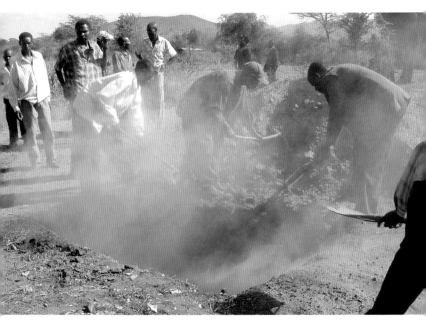

Funeral in Kithituni

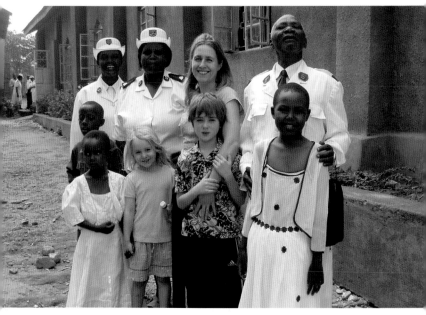

Salvation Army, Kithituni, including:
Margaret, Major Grace, Agnes, Nicola, Gabriel and Jonathan

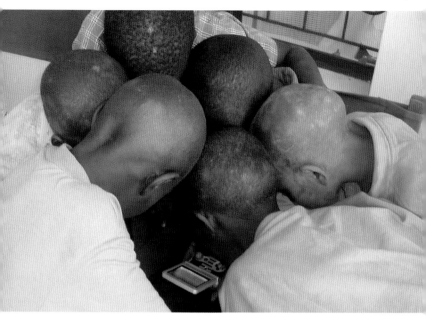

Gameboy!

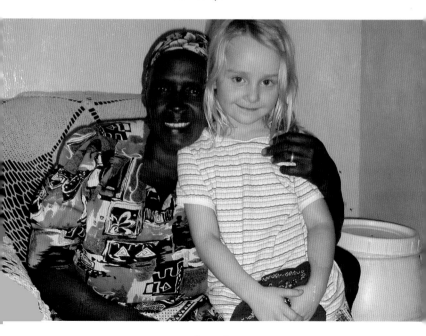

Big Agnes with Little Agnes

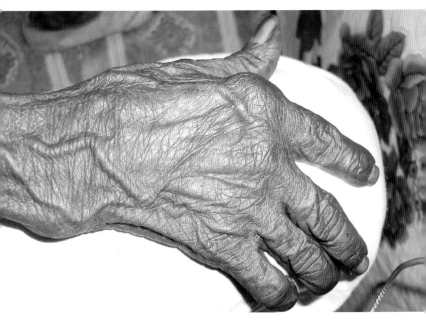

Mama Safi's hand

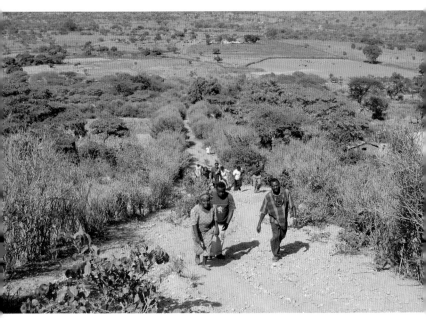

The Kithituni team out on a home visit

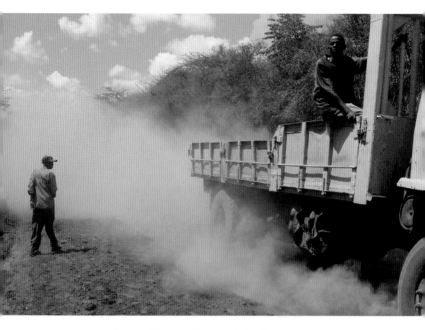

The sand-boys off to work, Kithituni

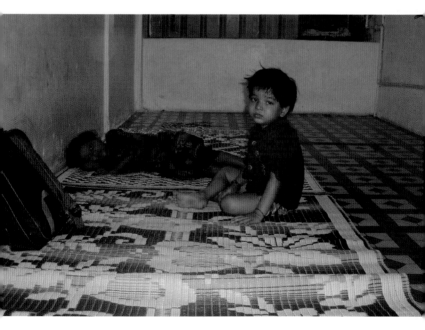

Children of sex-workers at the drop-off centre, Mumbai, India

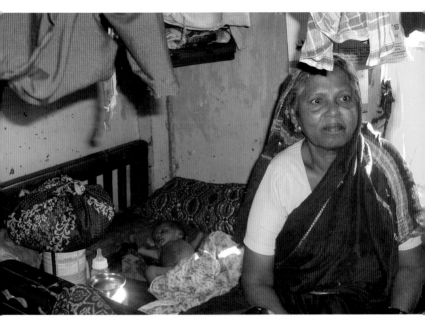

A Madam and a two-week-old baby in a Mumbai brothel, India

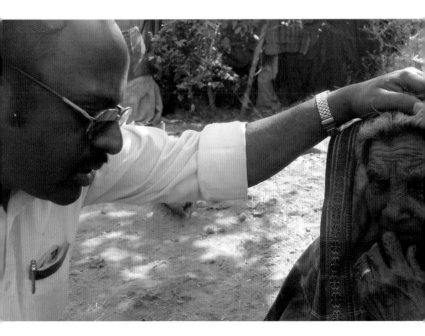

Major Randive prays for a woman in the street, Satara, India

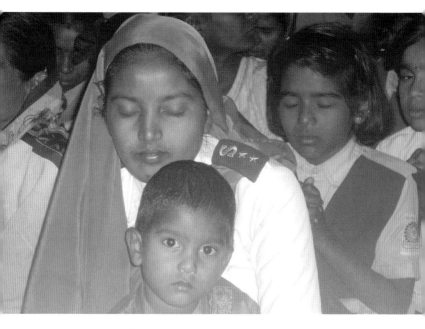

A Salvation Army officer at worship

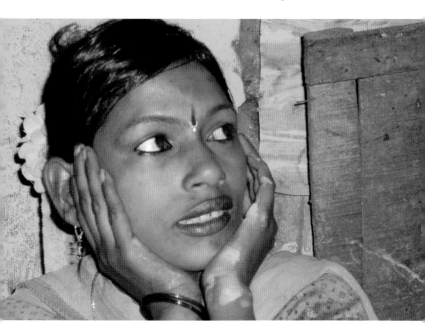

A fifteen-year-old prostitute, Satara

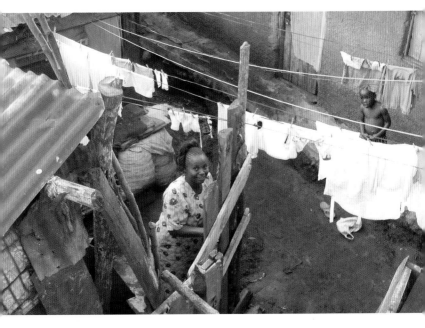

The Kibera, Nairobi, Kenya

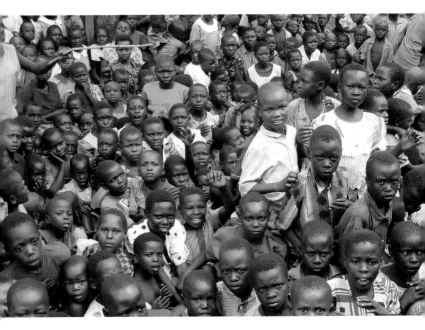

In the field of a thousand orphans, Uganda

but even a thorough search for answers to this question had led the author Philip Gourevitch – who spent two years in the country – to a place of confoundment. He concluded that even when you stack up the explanations to the point where genocide seemed inevitable, a logical outcome of circumstance and event, when it finally happened the killing had been utterly gratuitous. The more explanations I read – overpopulation, poverty, two rival tribes, a heritage of colonial manipulation – the harder it was to answer the why question. None of these fully explained why so many people killed their neighbours in such a way and on such a scale. They didn't explain what goes through the mind of a man raising a machete to hack off the limbs of his neighbour's son or through the mind of a man raping his neighbour's wife. And perhaps that's because genocide really requires a hidden change in the mind for it to become a reality; maybe a blanking out of self, some emptying of humanity that can't be detected until it's too late.

In trying to reduce tremendous happenings to a checklist of digestible, manageable 'facts', things get left out. And maybe this is why we never learn from history: history accounts for the big, seen, usually noisy, recordable events but leaves out the inner workings of men's hearts and minds; the dead, dull void that is necessary for a man to do appalling things doesn't make the manuscripts of record because, like the hidden acts of kindness, it cannot always be recorded.

I was already leaving things out.

'It was about one tribe of people fighting the other.' I said.

'Did one tribe come from another country?' Gabriel asked.

'They were living in the same country, often neighbours and sometimes friends.'

My son thought about this for a few seconds. 'How could they be friends and kill each other?'

'They were told lies about their friends. And they believed the lies.'

'That's dumb,' he said.

Major Florence Malabi and her husband Major Joash met us at Kigali International Airport. They embraced us warmly and we greeted them with our limited Kiswahili. The Malabis were Kenyans and their faces lit up at the sound of this *muzungu* family speaking their native tongue (it doesn't take much for foreigners to please people – just a 'hello' or a 'how are you?' in their language and a friendship is established).

Florence and Joash had been posted here two years before and were effectively the Territorial Commanders, responsible for overseeing the Army's activity throughout the whole country. Rwanda was a relatively new territory for the Salvation Army. They had been here just twelve years – since the genocide. After the first officers arrived in 1994 to assist in providing humanitarian aid, they were registered as an NGO in 1995 and then as a Church in 2003. A relatively small band they punched well above their weight. And they needed to. A look at the activity they were engaged in gave a fair inventory of the issues faced by this incredibly damaged, needy nation: clean water projects; house building; poverty alleviation projects: child sponsorship, 'the upliftment' of women, emergency feeding; as well as self-reliance training and community capacity building. Without the genocide Rwanda would have been a priority territory for any corps; with it, it was front line.

The greatest challenge faced by the Salvation Army here – indeed by any agency trying to help – was dealing with the psychological legacy of the genocide. Rwanda had many visible, tangible needs and as many practical responses, but the great unseen was the damage done to people's minds and emotions – to their spirit. It was twelve years since the genocide, but the collective shock of those events was – as we were to discover – still in evidence.

Kigali was a quiet, beautifully set city that felt like a peaceful, rural town. There was a lively bustle about the streets where the people were going about their day, visiting market, catching a bus, going to school. Its low-rise architecture didn't feel like the concrete, Western sprawl of Nairobi; it was sedate, almost refined. It actually seemed to have a greater sense of a culture and an identity. And the country had great roads, roads that, unlike Kenya's, remained great all the way to the farthest borders – Burundi, Congo and Uganda.

Our new home was a two-hour-drive north of Kigali, in a village settlement in Kayenzi District. Joash and Florence accompanied us there. Florence – a shrewd and kind woman – explained the itinerary she had prepared for us. We were to stay with a young Salvation Army couple – Captain Celestine and Beatrice and their two children – for the first week. And then with another Salvation Army couple – Nicodeme and Janvier and their children – in a nearby district, for the second. Both couples were Rwandan. They had a little English but if we could speak French that would help. They would be able show us the work there and help understand the AIDS situation.

As we drove out of Kigali and into the hills, the view from our passing car presented the familiar African pageant of colour and movement: women in coloured print skirts, balancing all manner of produce on their heads and often with a baby strapped to their back; young men in football shirts – usually Arsenal or Chelsea (two teams with a high quota of French speaking Africans) – riding bikes made in China at breakneck speed up and down the undulating ridges. To my eye it all looked no poorer than anything we had encountered in Kenya or India; in fact, the green glow and pastoral activity really created the impression of fruitfulness, of plenty. Later we'd see, close up, that the agricultural activity in the stripped forest slopes had a haphazard, frenzied quality born of too many people in too small an area trying to cultivate food for too many mouths.

I asked Joash how we would be received by the people.

Guessing the subtext of my question, Joash said we would be safe; but because the people were not used to seeing a *muzungu* family in these parts that we should be ready for people to stare. This surprised me. I had imagined Rwanda to be so full of foreign NGOs and aid workers since the genocide that the people would be used to seeing foreign people but there were not that many visitors outside of the city, except those who had come specifically to see the mountain gorillas in the north of the country.

Once we came off the main road and onto the track that took us to Kayenzi we could see those volcanoes, running like a row of jagged teeth to the north, the peaks of the tallest shrouded in the mist that had made them and their rare inhabitants famous. For a time after the genocide the gorillas remained unseen by visitors; but the treks were now well and truly back; so popular that the gamekeepers were getting concerned that the gorillas were being exposed to too many people. People paid up to two thousand US dollars a head to see them. They flew into Kigali, checked into a hotel, took a jeep to a lodge in the mountains, did the trek and then returned, without ever once stepping from the tourist trail to engage with the humanity that was all around them. It is a common problem in African countries blessed with amazing wildlife. People fly in, live in a bubble of comfort and sanitised adventure, a micro-economy that is expensive even by Western standards; they see some animals and then leave, having made little connection with the indigenous population. In Rwanda this is something of an achievement as the population is never made sparse by vast tracts of land. It is the most densely populated country in Africa (by the year 2020 it is estimated it will double, to about eighteen million) with 272 inhabitants per square kilometre. When we came off the main road and headed through the settlements, further into the countryside, the amount of people milling around didn't diminish. It seemed to increase.

Despite Joash telling us we would be safe, I didn't feel totally reassured. The complicit involvement of so many people in the genocide was so total; you knew that most of the people you were seeing had either perpetrated acts of murder or witnessed scenes so damaging that the only people who might be free of the scars were those aged twelve and under. Add to this the images gleaned from the newsreel and films about this country's recent history and it was almost impossible not to look upon everything through a prejudiced prism.

In a short, two-hour-journey I caught myself thinking:

'Isn't that the street where people were hacked down by the Interahamwe?* That man has a scar. Probably from a machete. President Juvénal Habyarimana's plane was shot down there as a signal to start the genocide.'

And although everyone – from President Paul Kagame to the Major and his wife – had a self-imposed embargo on mentioning Tutsi or Hutu (they were all Rwandans now) it was impossible not to see the differences between the taller, lithe, high cheek boned Tutsis and the shorter, squatter, wider faced Hutu.

After a while, I told myself to stop it. We weren't going to see much or learn anything being this paranoid. The only way to kill fear was to engage with the people.

That night, tucked up in our new home, we were woken by a scream. It was the scream of a woman although it was so primal that we thought it might be an ape or some tropical bird. I think I wanted to believe it was an animal rather than a person. After the scream, there was silence and then a continuous, low moaning; the sound of someone in pain. The woman was muttering words in between the groans. There was no other sound. No sense of anyone helping or attacking her. And it all sounded close, as if she were just outside the house gates, right in the road.

---

* A Hutu paramilitary youth group whose name means 'those who stand together'.

We lay there, wondering what was happening: was she having a baby? Had she just been attacked, or raped? The speculation and the lack of an answer escalated my thoughts: perhaps she was some kind of witch-doctor come to establish her territory. Or maybe she had been awoken from a dream made from memories of what had happened to her, or what she had seen, or what she had done herself.

Dare we get up and see if she was alright?

Eventually we could hear the voices of Captain Celestine and the night guard and see a torch-light beam investigating at the gates. It was hard to make out what he was seeing but after that there weren't any more sounds. The night returned to silence; a silence that was striking for it really being a silence. In India we had been kept awake most nights by continual dog barking. Here in Rwanda there were hardly any dogs because they had been shot during the genocide to stop them eating the bodies of the massacred and spreading infection. A film about the genocide – *Shooting Dogs* – was being screened in Kigali later that month and had taken its name from this phenomenon. Months later, when we were back in England, we would see this film about a gap year student 'doing his bit for Africa' caught up in the genocide; in the film the student befriends a Catholic priest who when given the chance of escape refused to leave his 'flock' and ended up being hacked to death with his congregation in the church. The student, unlike the priest, decided not to stay, to get out while he could.

After the incident of the screaming woman in the night, I found it hard to sleep; hard not to think about the screaming that must have filled the air twelve years ago during those horrific hundred days, hard not to think about a country in which there was no hiding place from evil – not even in a church.

I knew I would have got out if I could.

Captain Celestine, Beatrice and their two boys had given up their bedrooms to accommodate us and were sleeping in the hut next to the pit latrine. At breakfast we expressed concern; had they been comfortable and warm enough? The nights were cool now and damp. This was the season of the short rains (they were late this year) and it was the time of year where the change in temperature and moisture caught people out and gave them colds. I had noticed that Beatrice had a cough and was struggling a little; but she gave a very jovial reply.

"Yeeees!' she said. 'Fiiine.'

She had this sing-song inflection that remained consistent, whatever the subject. Only later, when I would feel comfortable enough to ask her about her own experiences during the genocide, did her voice lose its brightness as she told me about her father refusing to leave his village and being killed.

When we asked about the noise in the night Celestine nodded and gave a nervous laugh. He shook his head. He seemed more annoyed than worried. This woman, whoever she was, had made a scene before.

'What was wrong with her? It sounded bad.'

But Celestine seemed not to know − or unable to explain in English − so we remained in the dark.

We ate a breakfast of burned toast (fried in a pan without oil), the honey we had bought in Kigali, tea, banana and pineapple. The houseboy brought porridge, slightly burned, and then more burned toast. Lunch and dinner would be equally imposing and the portions just as grand. For all the talk of it being poorer than its larger neighbour, Kenya, Rwandans seemed to enjoy a greater variety of produce: potatoes, cabbage (made into coleslaw) pineapple, banana, and slightly less scrawny meat. Only after a week did we begin to notice the staples recurring.

Breakfast was made and served by a housekeeper, a short, gentle man and a young mother who stirred the pots in the yard with a baby strapped to her back. It was common for Salvation Army officers to employ staff. Although for us the idea of having domestic help smacks of luxury this is not as grand as it sounds;

it had more to do with necessity than status. Female officers were expected to work as much as male, even if they had children; it was also a necessary way of creating employment and spreading the wealth around. A Salvation Army officer was paid very little but it was a regular income that came with accommodation and in a country where 69% of the population live on less than a dollar a day that equated to riches.

The amount of food we were served was almost embarrassing. Celestine, Beatrice and their sons ate copiously but we couldn't keep up. Africans – at least Kenyans and Rwandans – served huge portions of whatever it was that was available. They might go without a meal for a day or even two but when they ate they went for it, as if eating what was there while it was there. The demands (walking, lifting, carrying, digging) of an average African day required a big calorie intake. They were getting ready for the walking we were going to be doing later that day.

After breakfast, I tested Celestine on African capital cities from my *Lonely Planet* guide. He gave a correct answer to every question I asked him, including the capital of the Central African Republic (Bangui) – a country I didn't even know existed. I rated my geography general knowledge but my knowledge of African capitals was poor; I could name more American States than African countries.

Celestine and Beatrice's quarters lay on a ridge that over-looked the volcanoes and the Nyungwe Forest to the north. It was a view you could stare at for hours; Rwanda, Kenya, all the Africans countries we visited, were always pulling this trick of making you feel you were in a paradise; a sensation you could go with for as long as you kept your eyes fixed on the view rather than the daily struggles of the people.

But in all our time there we could never fully give ourselves to that panorama. People talk about there being a bad atmosphere, almost a curse upon places where terrible things have happened

– Auschwitz, Hiroshima, the Gulags. Rwanda was the first place I really felt this.

People stopped and stared at us staring at the landscape. They formed a semicircle, children at first, then adults. Women, balancing produce on their heads, making their way along the road to market, stopped and joined the gallery. It was hard to say what they found more curious: the fact that we were looking at the view, or the fact that we were a family of white people in a remote part of Rwanda with no tourist attractions. Our children were particularly fascinating; especially Agnes who was whiter and blonder and cuter than the rest of us. Several women touched and tried to take her hands. As the crowd grew a strange unease grew with it that I tried to dispel by engaging them in French. When we spoke they laughed and mimicked our accents. It is a myth that most Rwandans speak French. Paul Kagame, the Rwandan President, decided long ago that he couldn't be bothered to learn French. A decade ago only one in eight Rwandans spoke French, even though it was the official language. Now more and more people speak English. Some say this is because French is the language of oppression; and the language of genocide and death.

Agnes pulled away from the grabbing and hid behind me; there was more aggression than affection in these gestures; I raised a hand to deter them but the women continued to try and pull at her arms. Seeing the gathering crowd outside the compound encircling us, Captain Celestine dispersed them, clapping his hands as if shooing cattle and saying something to them I didn't understand. I felt disappointment. We were trying to be friendly, but we had failed to connect; something wasn't happening and it wasn't just a matter of lacking language. It was uncomfortable. I couldn't work out if their grabbing Agnes was just a cultural thing or something unhealthy let loose in them by recent events. This latter thought was compounded when we went to see the market and a man suddenly grabbed Agnes as if to steal her. Not sure of his intentions and not having time to assess them I yelled at him and pulled Agnes back from his grasp. He laughed at my reaction, as if to say he was only joking or it was nothing, and kept on going. We were a mere two hours from the capital city, an international centre with four star hotels and a university, and yet these people reacted to us as complete aliens with seemingly no reference points as to what planet we came from.

A group of men – aged between twenty and forty – sat on the veranda of the pub drinking banana beer, the common local brew in Rwanda; their loss of inhibition had them calling out for us to join them as we passed through the town on our way to visit the medical centre. Celestine commented that this is what many men in Rwanda did: they have no work or they do a little cultivation and then they drink. It was a stereotype you didn't want to believe, but with every village we passed through the stereotype was reinforced. Some say inebriation and drug use – mainly ghat chewing – is the cause of many of Africa's woes. In Rwanda, the Interahamwe had got drunk in order to carry out their atrocities. Drunk men are more likely to rape women, or sleep with someone for gratuitous pleasure; less likely to work, less likely to bring money home, less likely to love and support a wife and children; more likely to have and pass on HIV. The combination of a cheap and dangerously sedative brew, a lack of opportunity, and the time that they have on their hands that comes from that lack of opportunity does for many of them.

William Booth could so easily have been describing the roadside African scene when he wrote of the inebriated male, in *In Darkest England*: 'I will take the question of the drunkard, for the drink difficulty lies at the root of everything. Nine tenths of our poverty, squalor, vice and crime spring from this poisonous tap-root. Many of our social evils, which overshadow the land like so many upas trees, would dwindle away and die if they were not constantly watered with strong drink…the loss which the maintenance of this huge standing army of men who are more or less always besotted men whose intemperance impairs their working power, consumes their earnings, and renders their homes wretched, has long been a familiar theme…'

Meanwhile, while the men don't, the women do and so another African (maybe a Developing World) cliché takes form before our eyes: women holding it all together, doing the work, raising the children, farming the land, feeding the family; while the men, still believing in some quasi chief-like role for themselves, sit around. Some call this the Big Boss mentality: a corrupted, deformed tribal hang over. But these days, you don't have to be a great man to acquire it. Others say, it is a cultural practice exacerbated by lack of opportunity.* Booth had another theory that made sense to me:

> '…lectures against the evil habit are, however, of no avail. We have to recognise that the gin palace…although poisonous, is still a natural outgrowth of our social conditions. The tap-room in many cases is the poor man's parlour. Many a man takes to beer, not from the love of beer, but from a natural craving for the light, warmth, company and comfort which is thrown in along with the beer…and which he cannot get except for buying beer.'

Why, though, could a man not get the light, warmth, company and comfort he needed without having to seek out drinkers? Was no one else offering him these things?

At the medical centre we were greeted by the great, life-affirming sound of a hundred babies crying. The mothers of newborns in the district – there must have been over one hundred of them

---

* The Salvation Army offers a radical counter example to the role of men and women in society. The equality of status achieved between men and women in the Salvation Army, especially given the patriarchal cultures in which they operated, was one of the more radical things we encountered on the journey.

there – were here on this particular day to give their babies their inoculations against polio and TB. The place was buzzing. In the courtyard a weigh scale dangled from the rafters and a sister weighed a screaming babe and made a satisfied nod of approval. The baby was a good weight and it had a fully operational set of lungs.

The medical centre was clean and relatively well stocked but lacking in one key piece of equipment. I asked Beatrice: '*Où est le docteur?*'

Technically, this was not a hospital, it was a medical centre, so a doctor was not required. But many doctors had left Rwanda, or been killed during the genocide. There were said to be only 150 doctors in the entire country for eight million people.

Despite this dismal statistic it was impossible not to feel cheered by this place; new life was the best antidote to the morbid oppression of recent times.

Rwanda has one of the world's highest birth rates at 3.2% per annum. This is a mixed blessing. Beatrice explained that Rwandans had always had big families and that in the old days there had always been enough land, therefore food, therefore enough money to manage. Now this wasn't the case and women were being encouraged to have smaller families. This was easier said than done. It was men who called the shots around here and men were not considerate of long-term planning.

In Rwanda, AIDS was genocide's bastard offspring and it was the women and children who were the victims. There were an estimated 200,000 rapes during the genocide; rape by men carrying HIV was used as a deadly, far-reaching weapon of war. Of the 200,000 rapes, 100,000 were infected. Of the 260,000 orphans, 65,000 were HIV positive. And of the 100,000 Rwandans that now needed treatment only 4,000 were receiving antiretroviral treatment.

The nurse let me see the HIV testing book – the first I had been allowed to see – and it was a most telling document. It showed that, as well as the prevalence of HIV positive people in this district being about 6%, that it was mainly the women who were infected. This itself didn't tell the whole story because of course, true to form, it was the women who came for testing. Partly because they were all tested when they were pregnant, but also because they were more responsible about their bodies and about the possibility of contracting HIV/AIDS. I looked at the book – a list of 250 names – and there were only five men registered as having had an HIV test. Men drank banana beer; women got tested.

Ahhhhhhhh! You wanted to scream. The men again. It was beginning to feel like this issue – men and their poor attitudes to sex, to families, to work, to testing, to wearing condoms, to women's sexual freedom and choice – lay at the root of more than just the problem of HIV/AIDS. It was a kind of sub-pandemic all on its own.

Walking back home, Beatrice sang a hymn in French. I put it to her.

'You know what the big problem here is – in Rwanda, maybe in the whole of Africa, maybe the world? It is the men. The men need help. I mean…where are the men?

Où sont les hommes!

Beatrice laughed knowingly. 'Yeeesss! Where are the men?'

The genocide has so dominated the mental landscape and thinking in Rwanda that it has superseded all other problems, even AIDS. A friend of mine who spent several months in Kigali researching a paper on violence, commented that in his whole time in Rwanda he hardly ever met anyone with AIDS, a comment that astonished me at the time. Part of this problem was actually connecting with the people. In Rwanda this was much harder to do. Getting people to talk about AIDS was always a challenge in itself; but with the horrors of genocide complicating things, there was a double taboo to be surmounted. Beatrice, through patient visits and making connections, had tried to break though these things. Her view was that if people were going to meet to talk about the one then perhaps they might talk about the other. Because of rape, they usually went together.

After the hospital visit Beatrice took us to meet a woman – Alphonsene – who had lost all her family in the genocide, been raped by the Interahamwe and made HIV positive in the process. High cheek-boned and calm, wrapped in the colourful shawl favoured by the Rwandese women, Alphonsene was a striking figure. She had a heavy demeanour but it was hard to match this woman to the story of the things done to her. What was all the more astonishing was that she was now leading the HIV/AIDS response team in Bagoma district. To do that she not only had to share her story, she had to sit with relatives of people who had done nothing to save her.

We talk of forgiveness and we subscribe to the theory of forgiveness, but this was what it looked like in the flesh.

Later we visited a mother – Marie Rose – and her three children Marie Claire, Blaise and Innocent. Her husband was in Kigali collecting the ARVs that she and her son needed to take (not all men were wasters). Again, the medical centre, because it lacked a doctor, was unable to distribute ARVs and so people (usually sick, poor people) had to travel two, three hours to the city to get them (they were trying to change the legality of who dispensed ARVs to get round this problem). Both Marie Claire and her son were HIV positive. The eldest child had been born before she was infected and the youngest whilst she was taking ARVs. Marie Claire's situation was almost the archetype for the pernicious cycle that AIDS creates for poor families: she was trying to run a home; she was too weak to cultivate crops with which to feed her family; and the medicine she needed was too far away for her and required her husband to travel and spend money they didn't have to get them. It wasn't for want of money; it was a simple problem of distribution.

Marie Rose's house was more elegantly decorated than any Kenyan home I had seen. The Rwandans seemed to have a better sense of style, both in terms of dress and décor, than their neighbours. Her simple house had two rooms, sparely furnished, and with the light coming through the window and with the simple, wooden tables and chairs it felt like a home cared for and dignified. On the walls there were pictures of Jesus of the Sacred Heart, and a poster of an icon of Mary, suckling the infant Christ. Breast-feeding and AIDS. I tried not to think what I was thinking.

The fact that this family were Catholic clearly had no bearing on the AIDS response work that the Salvation Army were encouraging in this district. Faith, creed, race: it was irrelevant. I had read the mission statement (to minister to the whole person); here was the proof. AIDS was no respecter of man's little divisions and the response to it required people to break with traditions and former prejudices. Something bigger was at stake.

One day, I went for a walk to get away from the compound, to try and think about something other than genocide and AIDS or simply to not think at all. On the way I met an old couple, a husband and wife. They greeted me with such warmth – the first people in a week other than our hosts who had done this. Florence had told me that there was a whole generation who remembered what life was like before the genocide and although they had lived through terrible things they had retained some faith – in humanity, or God. It was the young who were wary and less likely to engage you in conversation – and so it proved. This couple bore themselves differently, not just because of age. As I pointed to the volcanoes in the far distance and mumbled a superlative in French they nodded in agreement and thanked me for the compliment, taking it to be a personal blessing.

Later, I was standing still looking at the view of the volcanoes and listening to music on my iPod (something I had not done until now) when a battered old Renault pulled up next to me. The driver introduced himself as Father Philip. He was in his sixties, maybe older, and he spoke good English with a thick, Hispanic accent. Father Philip asked what I was listening to. I offered him my headphones.

The old priest's head began to move to the pounding drive of the music – a piece of chamber music by the French composer Marin Marais. Father Philip smiled, enjoying and appreciating it. 'This is good,' he said. He said he liked to listen to music like this when he could but it was not easy because his radio reception of the BBC World Service was not good.

I explained that I was doing some broadcasts for the BBC World Service and that I was here with my family, staying with the Salvation Army. When I said Salvation Army he immediately made the connection with Celestine and Beatrice. They had once been members of his congregation before joining the Salvation Army. Without any rancour he said that many people had started leaving his church and going to the Salvation Army church. He added that they were good people. He had lived in Rwanda for forty years.

Talking to him immediately made me realise how deprived of a certain kind of conversation I had been and I wanted to talk to him more. I asked him if he would come to the compound and talk and he agreed.

When I told Celestine and Beatrice that Father Philip was coming to talk to me I sensed hesitation – certainly in Celestine. Churches, like NGOs and Aid agencies, can get very competitive and protective of their patches; I wondered if they saw him as a rival. I told them that Father Philip had acknowledged the good work of the Salvation Army here and seemed not to begrudge them their success in attracting new members; Beatrice said they knew him well, that he had been helping the people for years now and was a good man.

Father Philip came on time and he was received by Celestine and Beatrice with a certain formal decorum. It was interesting to see how Celestine and Beatrice treated him. They were like army officers deferring to naval officers in wartime. When it came to saying grace for our tea and biscuits it seemed in the natural order of things that the priest would say it.

To me they had more in common than not. The Salvationist and the Catholic might theologically speaking be distant members of the same family; in practice, they were often close neighbours, the only two Churches or organisations of any description to be found doing the work in the more remote and needy parts of the world.

Father Philip had opinions that many would consider to go against the perceived hard-line Catholic view (no contraception, a preference for large families and an urgency to see infants baptised).

When I asked him to tell me what Rwanda was like now and what were the most serious issues the people were facing he immediately said: overpopulation. People were having too many children and the lack of family planning or freedom that women had to plan was a serious issue.

'Poverty is getting worse now,' he said, 'because the low people (he meant poor people) were having too many children. They should have fewer children.'

When I said it was unusual to hear such a thing from a Catholic priest he said, 'I use my eyes. The girls and boys are becoming desperate. There is not enough land, work, school; they cannot have these families any more.'

This wasn't some unorthodox heresy being perpetrated by a renegade priest; it was simply a view born out of forty years of practice in the field; praxis over exegesis.

'So how can they deal with the problem of overpopulation?'

His answer was unequivocal.

'Give women freedom.'

'But that needs the men to cooperate and they're pretty unhelpful.'

'We need to teach – everyone, the schools, the church, we need to teach healthy sexual relations between man and wife.'

'Abstinence is not enough?'

'Abstinence is not real. Tell people not to do something – like sex – and they will do it; like Eve and Adam eating the apple.'

'So people need to talk about the apple. Talk about sex?'

'Yes. We must talk about these things.'

I then asked him if we could talk about something else that was hard to talk about. The genocide. I said it had been very hard to talk about this. It was as if people were too ashamed to talk about it.

'Yes,' he said. 'They are "shame-ed"' and the word with his accent sounded like the right word. Shame-ed. 'Here, in this area, seven hundred Tutsi were killed. And now there is shame. And still fear. But everyone suffer-ed. Tutsi suffer-ed, Hutu suffer-ed. Many Hutu die because they saved Tutsi. Before they were loving each other.'

'So what happened. What do you think is at the root?'

'It was easy to put genocide thinking in the people. Like Goebbels – with the German people. This is easy to do with the low people. This is why education is important.'

'And what happened to you during this time?'

Father Philip sighed deeply and his eyes filled with tears.

'We were all told to leave the country because it was dangerous. And they were killing priests. But I am unhappy because I left these people. I was not brave enough to stay. I went. To Burundi. That same day the gospel lecture was the shepherd and the lost sheep; the story about the good shepherd, risking his life for his sheep. I did not do. When I returned half my congregation were dead.'

His words and this image hung in the air for a few seconds. I wanted to say something, to lighten the old man's burden of guilt:

it was understandable. It was an extreme situation. What could he have done? But such words were of no consolation to a man whose job – at least in theory – was to look after and if necessary die for the people he served. I kept these thoughts to myself; I knew they were the platitudes of a man who would surely have got out himself had he found himself in the same situation.

I asked him how as a priest and a follower of Jesus he was able to preach a gospel of reconciliation and forgiveness in the light of all that his hearers had experienced. He thought for a moment and then said:

'As well as forgiveness I have to speak about justice. I have to speak about justice and forgiveness…'

'But this is a lot to ask of people.'

'Yes. But it is easier when you understand that God forgave everything before we even asked Him. Forgiveness is not an act of the intellect or even of the heart; it is an act of will – you have to choose it if you want to move on. In scripture it says God not only forgives our transgressions, He forgets them. But this is hard for men to do.'

For my birthday we decided to go into Kigali and celebrate with a day at the *Hôtel des Mille Collines*, the capital's best hotel and famous for being the actual hotel in the film *Hotel Rwanda*. This book-ending of stays in remote, uncomfortable places was something that helped keep the spirits up (we had done it in Mumbai and Calcutta and would do it wherever we could); but it was never totally comfortable; it always felt like a cheat, going from pit latrine to porcelain bidet; from coleslaw to roquette and focaccia. How easy it is to switch from lack to largesse and back again.

We caught a bus into town, our exotic presence causing more mirth among the passengers. The bus driver cranked up the radio that was pumping out a pretty lively Afro-pop that we all jiggled our legs to. Suddenly I realised that the song we were listening to was about Arsenal Football Club. The recurring lyric at the end of the verse being 'Arsene Wenger, Arsene Wenger', the name of the club's French manager. The song then went into a litany of reasons for the club's greatness. The song, sung in Rwandese was currently in the country's top ten. The ubiquity of football throughout Africa had this slightly misleading normalising effect on the mind of (European) visitors. Like the landscape and the wonderful wildlife, it made you think things were fine after all; but the music did make me think if these people can sing a song about Arsenal then surely their minds are on lighter, brighter things. Paul Kagame did cite the increase of the numbers of people playing and watching football as a sign that things were returning to normal. Sport, he said, was one way of taking people's mind off heavy things.

The hotel was a modern, pleasant L-shaped, seven-storey building built around a swimming pool and tennis courts and set in a terraced garden. The clientele was largely black and, according to the waiter, Rwandan; elegantly dressed businessmen and women sat drinking bottled beer and Perrier discussing things. Waiters served people who sat at tables poolside. This was where, during the Genocide, the then hotel owner, Paul Rusesabagina, opened up his hotel to both Tutsi and Hutu refugees and then, using bribes and favours he had built up as manager of the hotel and blackmailing a corrupt general, he managed to save the lives of 1,268 refugees. It was hard to imagine this place being sanctuary to a thousand people fleeing for their lives but this was where that particular drama – now re-enacted and committed to celluloid – had been played out.

At the bar I met a young American who was a doctor, specialising in infectious diseases – HIV/AIDS in particular – studying at Princeton and here in Rwanda doing groundwork. We got talking and he explained that he was actually based in Kampala, but had come to Rwanda on assignment. Because he was American and a doctor working with AIDS I asked him if he had read a book called *Mountains Beyond Mountains* by Tracy Kidder. The book was about a brilliant doctor, Paul Farmer, who had a radical approach to healthcare that involved what he called 'preferential option for the poor.' Farmer's philosophy (theology, really) was that you should give the poorest people a standard of healthcare you would expect to provide for the rich, no matter what it cost. Acutely aware of how inequitably money and medical care are distributed in the world, Farmer argued that the only antidote for the 'structural violence' that keeps the poor too sick to climb out of the hole they are in is to treat health care as a basic human right and do whatever it takes to deliver it. Farmer had practiced in Haiti, deliberately seeking out the poorest places, within the poorest places, in order to practice, and he had recently come to Rwanda. His inspiration drew on the text, from Matthew 25 ('What you did to the least of these you did for me'), a scripture I would see written up, often laid out in the shape of a cross, in many Salvation Army churches.

The America doctor smiled and looked at me, slightly amazed. 'I have just sent a message to him, via an email. I was trying to meet him.'

'That's amazing. I was hoping to meet him myself.' And I explained a little of why.

Before the journey I had actually thought to try and connect Farmer with the Salvation Army's Dr Ian Campbell, who had himself pioneered a particular approach to healthcare through his work at Chikankata Hospital in Zambia. Farmer's approach and the Salvation Army's AIDS response work had some similar traits: they both went against conventional wisdom, involved family and friends and prioritised the poorest people. In Farmer's model, every AIDS or TB patient is assigned a paid health worker, or *accompagnateur* – generally a friend, relative or neighbour – who handled the drugs and made sure they were taken on schedule. The regional response teams we had worked with were effectively trying to do the same thing, the only real difference being that no one was paying them and they had no medical training. Farmer's approach seemed to be the missing link in the regional team's armoury: supplying the medical know-how; and the regional team's approach had what Farmer's approach could use a bit more of: a belief in people's capacity to do it themselves rather than you doing it for them.

It was a long shot, but meeting this doctor had me suddenly excited. Maybe there was some intended meeting that I had some part in brokering. But my American doctor friend had had no luck. 'I don't think he's here. He's always to-ing and fro-ing. Right now I think he is back in the States.' The two of us swapped email addresses and said we'd get in touch if either of us had any joy finding the great man.

We decided to take a vehicle down to the south, to Cyangugu, a town on the border with the Democratic Republic of Congo; to see something of the country and visit the prison there. To do this we had to hire a driver and vehicle (there was no car hire in Rwanda). Our driver was also called Celestine. He was a beautiful looking man, with several scars on his face. He had no English or French and the lack of communication on the long, winding drive south added to his mystery. The scars on his face were too random, too ill-placed to be anything decorative, tribal.

We travelled to Cyangugu Prison with Ainea Kimaro of the Kigali Institute of Science and Technology. I had been given Ainea's name by my friend Sarah Butler Sloss, the patron of the Ashden Awards, a charitable trust that rewarded innovative projects that tackle climate change and poverty and improved quality of life by providing renewable energy at a local level. Ainea's biogas installation at Cyangugu prison had won first prize.

Ainea was from Tanzania and spoke good English. As we drove he explained to us how his biogas plant worked. By capturing the methane from the raw sewage for cooking gas, and using the residue for fertiliser on crops to feed the prisoners, Ainea's invention had dealt with two big problems in one – creating a sustainable power and food supply. Since the genocide, thousands of people had been imprisoned in overcrowded jails, some packed with as many as ten thousand inmates. That meant huge numbers of meals to cook, sewage to treat and wood to burn, and Rwanda could ill afford to burn more wood. Even as we drove, we could see now the effects of soil erosion, caused through the felling of trees all throughout the country; this in turn affected the ability of farmers to grow sufficient crops. The seasons were changing, the rains less reliable – or the rains hardly ever came at all.

There it was again: climate change. Everywhere we travelled we met people who, without prompting, had talked about the weather changing: either too much rain (Mumbai), not enough rain (Kithituni) or utterly unpredictable rain (Rwanda). If for us – in the rich north – it was an urgent talking point, for many people in the countries we visited it was already catastrophic and having an immediate impact on all areas of life.

The prison was a rectangular, red brick fortress, overlooking Lake Kivu. This was a place where the complicated, flawed process of man's justice slowly works itself out. The five thousand inmates at Cyangugu prison all wore pink uniforms. Such a knowing colour that it must have been chosen for a reason. Was it to make them look foolish, or to emasculate them? We couldn't work it out, until my son said he thought it helped you to see them as people rather than murderers.

'It helped make you think of them as innocent,' he said.

I wanted to believe this observation. Many of these prisoners are, twelve years later, still yet to face trial. Most would have been boys at the time of the genocide, boys not much older than my son. The Gacaca system – where you gain your freedom if you confess your crime – was helping to speed up the process but this system was open to abuse, with prisoners making disingenuous confessions in order to be released, or genocidaires returning to their communities to commit revenge attacks on those who had testified against them. The director of the prison told me that it would take five years for these local courts to solve the back-log.

After viewing the biogas plant, the director let us see the entrance to the prison. We were not permitted inside the prison proper; this glimpse was intended to help us see that conditions were humane. Inside a courtyard about thirty or more prisoners lay in cells – cages really – some with as many as eight in one. We passed through quickly; whatever these people had done, it felt like a cruel taunt to walk by like this; like staring at animals in a zoo, and it was relief to exit the place.

Driving back to Kigali we plucked up the courage to ask Celestine our driver about the scars on his forehead. When we asked, he smiled and said he was in the army fighting the insurgents. Which army?

'RPF.'

This means he'd have fought in the army under the future President, Paul Kagame, who was then a general. As a soldier our driver would have seen people killed and most likely killed people himself. It was strange to think that we had entrusted our safety to a man who had probably done terrible things, but by now we were getting used to holding these possibilities in tension. It was actually the only way to proceed. Mistrust – however reasonable – was another form of unforgiveness and a block to rehabilitation. President Kagame had said himself in an interview with Gourevitch that there was no alternative to believing that people can change because they have been given a second chance. When pushed as to whether killers could be re-integrated into society he said 'I think you cannot give up on that – on such a person. I am sure that every individual, somewhere in his plans, wants some peace, wants to progress in some way.'

Beatrice and Celestine were working in this spirit. Partly because it was fundamental to their beliefs; but also because it was utterly practical. They simply could not do the work without seeing each person as worthy of help. A home-based, communal response to the problem of AIDS could not wait for a willing, open and relatively healed community. The nature of the Army's work required – demanded really – a faith or belief that every single human being has the capacity to change; sometimes that would mean encouraging a man or a woman to visit a sick neighbour in his home, even if that same neighbour (or a relative of that neighbour) had once come to his house to kill them.

On our last day, we went to see the Kigali Genocide Museum. It was a hot, hazy day; too hot to spend very long looking at the gardens, where 250,000 people had been buried in mass graves. Inside we walked slowly towards the dark entrance not really sure we wanted to see whatever it was they were going to show us. My wife went ahead to vet the display for the children.

Part of the purpose of the museum was to try and explain the history and therefore the roots of the catastrophe. To shed some light on the dead, dull void. To answer the 'why?' question. As a starting point it explained how during Rwanda's colonial years the Belgians issued identity cards classifying most of the Rwanda population as either Hutu, who made up the majority, or Tutsi. It was a classic divide and rule system, (not dissimilar to the British manipulation of power between the tribes in Kenya). These same identity cards would later be used for the purpose of discrimination and murder.

We followed the unfolding story, pictures and text mounted on boards, supported with video displays, stepping inexorably closer towards the appalling, wondering how much the creators were going to sanitise; how much were they going to reveal. We walked on through the post independence struggles, the massacres of Tutsi, their exile in Uganda, the formation by those exiles of the Rwanda Patriotic Front and its armed wing the RPA which would one day return under the leadership of Paul Kagame, rallying the

Rwandans, among his men, Celestine, our driver, and a thousand others picking up the scars of war. And then the shooting down of Habyarimana's plane (by his own followers) setting in motion the genocide itself, the signal to the Hutu militia (Interahamwe) to begin the systematic, coordinated killing; fuelled up with banana beer and propaganda, they set to work.

I could already see, around the curve of the corridor, the next photographic installation, a body lying in a road. I looked at my children. They had already seen people with AIDS, funerals, met prostitutes. Why not this? Was it not another epidemic of death with the same root cause? It was real and it was true and I had to trust that they could handle truth. So far they had shown they could handle it better than me. We stepped into the room. A large photograph showed the inside of a church where hundreds of people lay dead. This was the church at Kibungo, in Eastern Rwanda, where many Tutsi were slaughtered after seeking sanctuary there. The cadavers that covered the floor were half clothed, half intact, but past decomposition. They had been left like this – as a memorial – so that people might see and believe what they were seeing.

My daughter clutched at my hand and my son grimaced and said what it was.

'That is disgusting.'

Just then Nicola entered the room from the direction we were heading.

'I think it's too much for them,' she said. 'Not the pictures, but the video stuff.'

'Aaarr?" Gabriel protested. 'Why?

I continued on into the story.

They say that what goes into the head stays with you forever. Of all the images that are presented – and they are utterly uncompromising – the one I knew would stick in my head was video footage of four or five men with machetes hacking at a man lying in the street in Kigali. This was real footage, shot on video, and it had such an odd choreography. It didn't look right, almost as if people really weren't designed to do this or capable of ever looking right doing it.

The striking thing about this memorial museum is its lack of pretension. It isn't straining through its design or beauty or austerity to match the depth and gravitas of the event it's recalling. It doesn't need to. It doesn't want you to remember the plinth or the statue or the cenotaph or the smart architectural design: it wants you to glimpse something of the total awfulness of what man can do at his worst and it succeeds in doing this. Memorials to human suffering cover the earth. I don't know if it means we care more than we used to, or if these memorials make the events they commemorate less likely to happen again. It's comforting to think of genocides or holocausts or massacres as unique, one off, never again events and the museums and memorials that commemorate them as somehow putting a full stop after that event; but as we left the museum we read the well-intentioned words: 'Never Again' knowing full well that genocide was happening again, right now, and in a country not that far away, a country where one day someone else – an architect or artist – would design and raise a monument.

We wanted to leave Rwanda with something other than the memory of this museum and the genocide. It had left us heavy and flat. We wanted a sense of hope but you can't fake that feeling. Rwanda doesn't make this easy for you.

Just before our departure Florence took us to meet the new cadets at the Salvation Army training centre. Florence was responsible for recruiting and training the new cadets over a period of two years. Many of them were young married couples. We sat beneath the shade of the jacaranda trees and ate lunch together and talked about their hopes and expectations. I think our own expectations were so low at this point that we were caught out by the enthusiasm and exactitude of these young Rwandans. The men – especially the men! – were full of hope. They talked about their desire to transform their damaged society; they were full of ideas; they had plans. It was perhaps the most encouraging encounter we had had for weeks; you could sense the stories that were going to get written once these cadets got out into the communities where they were going to be sent. Earlier in the week, Florence had said that it would take future generations to heal this country. Sitting there, listening to these young Rwandans, we caught a glimpse of that future and it looked good.

In the Field of a Thousand Orphans

'If you tolerate this, then your children will be next'
– The Manic Street Preachers

The chanting continued unbroken for ten minutes:

> *Ai-o Khwakusimile ai-o!* (beat, beat, beat);
> *Ai-o Khwakusimile ai-o!* (beat beat beat).*

We sat beneath a rudely constructed canopy of canvas and UNICEF truck tarpaulin, on wooden chairs reserved for the guests of honour and received this greeting from nearly a thousand children – most of them orphans – with a mixture of awe and embarrassment. We were surrounded by a wall of sound; a wall of sound and a wall of faces, with each little brick in the wall an orphan, all gathered in a field in the Kisekele community, in the district of Mbale, on the Ugandan border with Kenya: a community about the size of Barnes – the bit of London where I live – and a place where every one in four children had lost a parent to HIV/AIDS. The smiling, white-toothed, gingham-checked, hand-me-down T-shirted wall of abandoned noise, all heads and bodies pressed together, strained to get a better view of the visiting *muzungu* family who were already two hours late.

The local dignitaries filed in to join us beneath the canopy:

---

* A welcome song. '*Ai-o Khwakusimile Ai-o*' means 'we are happy to see you'.

councilmen, the chief and Church leaders: the men in safari style jackets, outsized suits and one in a garish Calvin Klein print shirt; the women in loud patterned, high sleeved, bunch-shouldered Victorian style dresses (gaudy and gauche after the refined elegance of the Rwandese). They looked like a tribe of people who had been stylistically duped by a myopic tailor. There was some 'who's who' re-arranging in the seats beneath the canopy as a few more councilmen arrived, and then an old man in a pink shirt and an outsized jacket stepped forward, raised his arms to the God he hadn't given up on yet and asked Him to bless them and us and this meeting. The whole crowd was quiet and heads were bowed; but I kept my eyes open, transfixed by the numbers of children and one boy in particular, perched at the tree's apex, looking straight at me, scrutinising me.

The event began with a song and dance of welcome, sung in a heavily accented broken English by about twenty children who marched down the path from the hills, their voices growing louder as they came closer until they eventually gathered in a semicircle in front of us and sang:

'Well a-come our dear visitors.
We are so happy to see you here.
Sitty down and listen to us.
KAY club is singing for you…Hello, hello!'

We were then treated to a forty-minute gala performance of songs and semi-musical testimonies, beginning with an educational poem that detailed the characteristics and course of the disease:

'HIV is result of AIDS. AIDS is killing all, young and old. It weakens the human body. It has killed many people in Uganda. Our homes are full of orphans. AIDS has no cure. To avoid AIDS, avoid bad sex. Avoid anal sex. Maintain virginity. AIDS, AIDS, AIDS. No one loves me. Be careful. You see me now: I don't have parents.'

I looked at my family – slightly ragged from our bus journey from Rwanda, and subsequent car ride here to this far side of Uganda, ten paces from the Kenyan border – and wondered if we were worth all the effort. We were low in humour, energy and will and facing a fabulous greeting from a thousand orphans who had been told of our coming weeks before. I had that feeling – a feeling I had many times on our travels (a feeling ultimately egotistical) – that we were going to disappoint. I could see Nicola thinking the same thing.

Inadequacy, it turns out, is the healthy and right response to such largesse. The feeling that I needed to perform, to provide something, was really a cousin to the wrong-headed mind set that so many people come here with: the mindset that thinks 'I can make a difference'; 'I have something to bring'; 'I have something to teach.' Standing there in a field with nearly one thousand orphans, watching and listening to their efforts, I eventually stopped worrying about what I was going to say to the gathered crowd when the man in the pink shirt asked me. Instead, I remembered another piece of advice I had been given by Dr Ian Campbell on the eve of the journey: it's not about you.

The feeling that I was going to disappoint also stemmed from the fact that there was an expectation of me bringing a video camera to 'make a documentary for the BBC'. It was true that I had originally intended to bring a camera with me, but after a few weeks of using it in Kithituni I abandoned it in favour of the mini-disc recorder that I was using for my BBC World Service radio reports. The camera was clunky and invasive and had the annoying side affect of changing people's behaviour into a performance; I was getting more candid, more authentic 'pictures' for radio than for television. But the message (sent from the goat-powered internet in Kithituni to the power-sharing,* restricted email of the Salvation Army's district officer in Kampala over six

* The River Nile is slowing from lack of rain and that this is affecting the hydroelectric power in Uganda.

weeks ago) had failed to get through. Just an hour before this 'meeting of a thousand orphans' we had been met by a crowd of about five hundred women in a church building who had also waited several hours for 'The man from the BBC' to arrive.

I explained this to Joseph Malakisi – the Salvation Army's coordinator for psycho-social support in the western district – why I had decided not to bring the camera. He was gracious, understanding my reasons, but he suggested I make a show of doing a recording and was relieved that my mini-disc recorder had a big, 'TV news style' microphone with which I could record the sounds and the voices of the people.

I recorded a great deal that day, holding the microphone in the air to catch the singing and the illustrative dramas of the women in the church; their stories of facing off the disease with small, income-generating projects; and then the songs, testimonies and poems of the orphans of the KAY Club (Kids and Youth Club) in the field of Kisekele. I feel churlish even expressing criticism of an event such as we witnessed in that beautiful valley near Mbale; but there was something mechanical about it all. The experience confirmed something my wife and I had begun to suspect the day we left life in the village in Kithituni and set out on the long road of visitation that had taken us to India, Rwanda and now here: namely, how much better it is to participate than to observe and how the observing changes when you're engaged with the thing you're observing. I had already recognised a type of this problem in the use of the video camera. Like electrons that change their behaviour the moment you begin to observe them, human beings also enact a kind of Heisenberg's Uncertainty Principle by changing the moment you start to film them, record them or even write down their words in a notebook. It makes accurate 'witnessing' a real challenge. The problem lessened when we lived for a period of time among a community; but the white-jeep, NGO style visit always had this cursory quality that left us feeling uncomfortable with ourselves and sceptical of the things

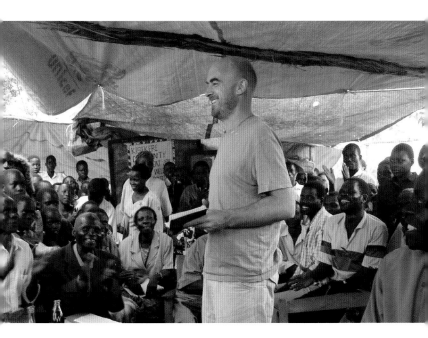

The author greets the gathering, Uganda

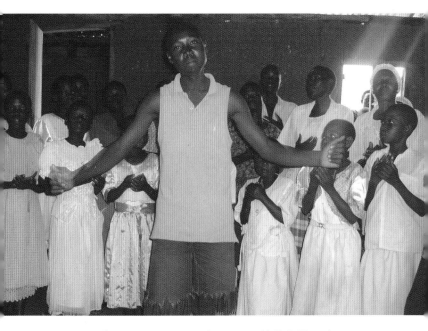

An orphan recites a poem about HIV/AIDS, Uganda

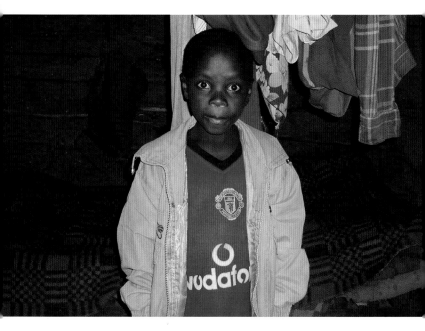

Patrick Nduati

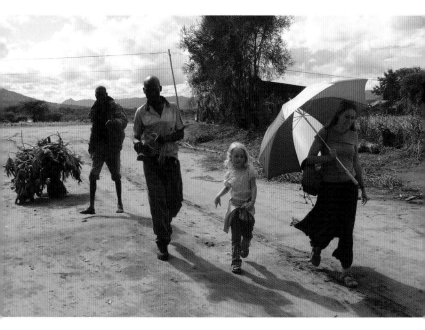

Nicola and Agnes returning from the market, Kithituni

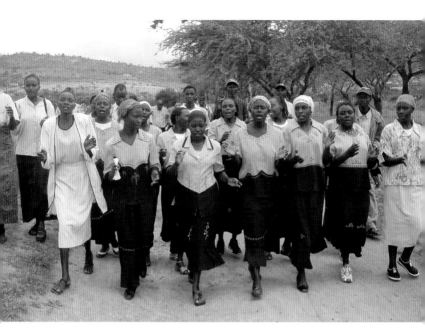

Greeting from the women near Machakos, Kenya

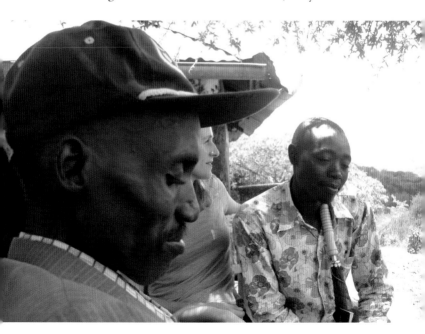

Pascal Kyengo

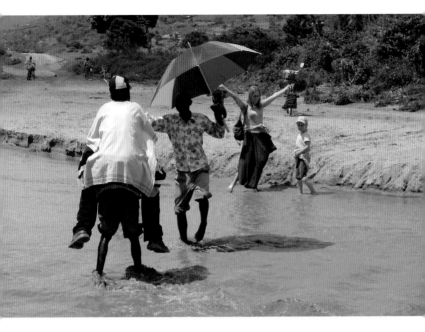

The rains have come, Kithituni

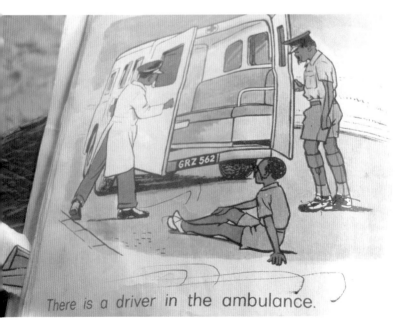

There is a driver in the ambulance.

Children's schoolbook, Zambia

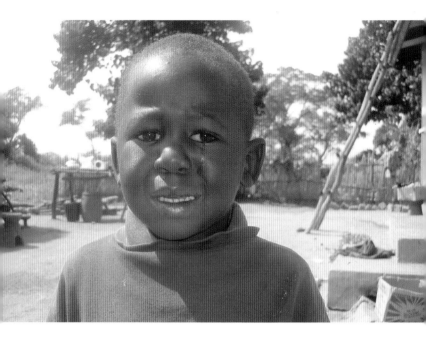

AIDS orphan, Zambia

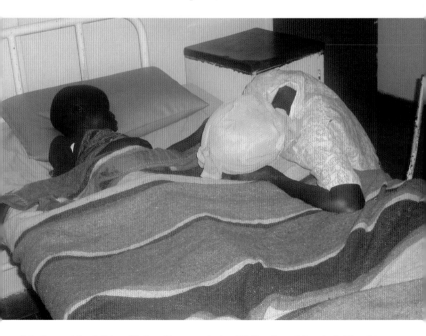

Mother with child suffering from malaria, Chikankata Hospital, Zambia

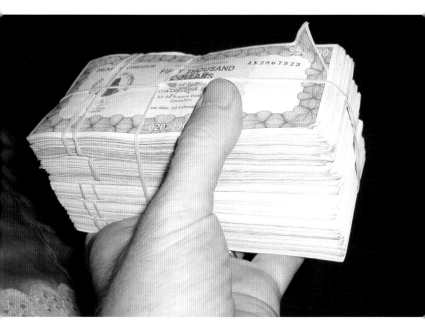

Inflation, Zimbabwe

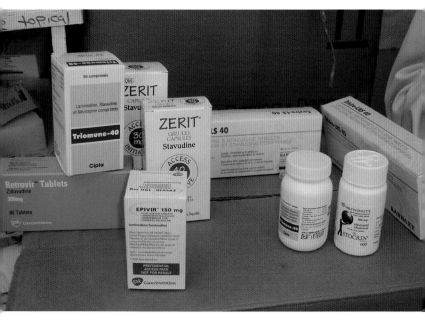

ARVs, Zimbabwe

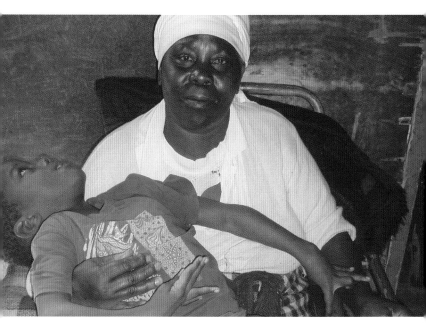

Grandmother with child, Soweto, South Africa

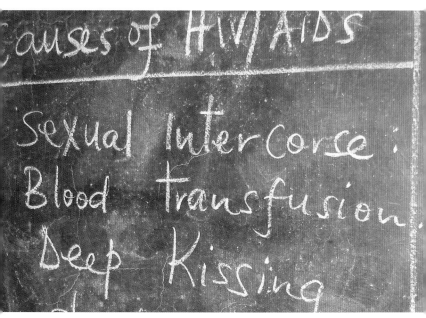

AIDS education, Uganda

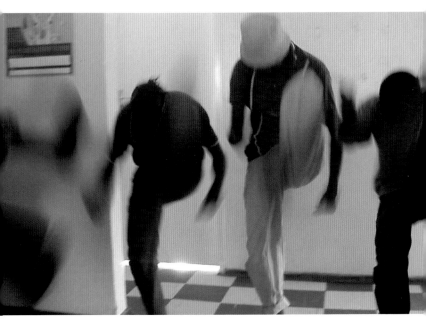

Orphans perform a Zulu dance, Soweto, South Africa

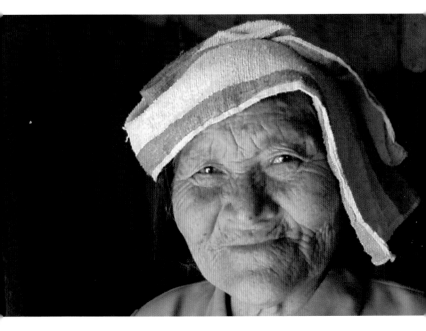

Farmer's wife, Henan Province, China

being 'presented'. You were constantly wondering how much of what you were encountering was performance, or an idealised summation of the things people wanted you to see and hear. Fleeting visits were necessary and sometimes the only way, but they never matched true engagement.

Some people describe HIV/AIDS as being like a wave that started in central Africa before passing southwards. In this sense, the disease had 'already passed through' Uganda, a country where the prevalence rate is now back down to 6% as compared to the rates in countries like Zimbabwe (25%) or South Africa (30%). Because of this fall, Uganda has been hailed as a good news story in the fight against AIDS, with the country being the first in Sub-Saharan Africa to see a decline in prevalence in the last few years. But statistics can be misleading (I would dearly loved to have written this book without including a single stat) and in the case of Uganda they have created a dangerous sense of 'having made it' – the consequence of which is a relaxation of effort. The decline in prevalence in Uganda was partly due to the quick and effective response efforts in the early years of the epidemic; but it is also due to the fact that Uganda has had among the largest number of deaths from the disease in the world, at around two million. Most of these were a particular generation – adults between the ages of 18 and 35 with children – which is why, everywhere we went, the number of children without parents seems so much greater than anything we had yet encountered. The lowering prevalence has been, in the main, down to the sheer numbers of people who have died. AIDS in Uganda has already killed a generation.

In Mbale we hired a Toyota Hyace minibus – a *matatu* – to get us to the communities on the border. I had the option of a four-wheel drive Jeep but I had the notion that driving a *matatu* would force us to engage more with people: after all, it could carry fourteen passengers (officially) and, if necessary, I would offer free lifts along the way. The *matatu* was also a reaction to having been chauffeured around in a mammoth Isuzu Trooper in Kigali (where there was no car hire) and not wanting to be seen in anything that might associate us with being an NGO (a specialised neurosis I was developing). Joseph was amused by my choice of transport. He said that I must be prepared for the van to be filled before we got to the village where we were going to stay. By the time we got there, we had 26 people and a chicken on board.

Along the way we were flagged down by a woman in distress. Her daughter was having a baby but there were complications: she needed a doctor. A vehicle this far out of town was a rare thing; ambulances didn't exist and this was an emergency. Our *matatu* was temporarily commandeered. The woman looked in pain as she was helped into the back. I drove as carefully as the roads would allow until we reached a town that had a medical centre and a doctor. I was half hoping she might have the baby in the *matatu*; but she hung on and had it that night, in the medical centre: a healthy boy.

I was told this the next day by Joseph on our way to another gathering (scaled down now after our conversation about finding it hard to connect in any meaningful way with groups of five hundred to a thousand a time).

'Do you know what they called the boy?' I asked.

He didn't know but he knew why I was asking. The woman had been told my name was Brook and there was an outside chance she might name the boy Brook – in honour of the willing *muzungu matatu* driver from London Town. Dr Ian Campbell had told me that many babies he delivered at the Chikankata Hospital in Zambia were called Doctor or Doctor Ian or even Doctor Ian Campbell by grateful mothers. Facilitating the birth of a child was a surefire and literal way of making a lasting name for yourself on this continent.

Joseph Malakisi was in his late forties. He had been working in the field of HIV/AIDS response for over ten years and for most of those ten years he had remained unpaid, getting by on donations and support from the Salvation Army. Now he received a small stipend, paid out of the PEPFAR (President's Emergency Plan for AIDS Relief) fund, the huge annuity donated by George Bush's administration. Joseph's role now was coordinator for pyscho-social support in the western region of Uganda. He was clearly good at what he did: those gatherings and the stories they had told – the kids club, the income-generating activity – would not have been possible without the community response that Joseph and April Foster had stimulated back in the 1990s. Their work was instrumental in changing the response to HIV/AIDS from being government driven to community-led.

To our eyes, what had happened – what we had been shown here – was some kind of a success story. But in the comments I had picked up on when I had interviewed Ian Campbell before the journey – comments backed by the regional response team back in Nairobi – there were reservations about PEPFAR and the influence big donors exercised on community response work. The reservations weren't about the conditions that sometimes came attached with such donations (ideological conditions) as much as the fact that money changes things. The general gist was that the funding could actually undermine the good work built up over years of diligent and committed interaction with the communities here because it changed the dynamic of how people worked. Once people got paid for responding to their neighbours' needs, so the argument went, something died. It was a classic case of money not necessarily being the answer.

This was a difficult thing to prove and the money a hard thing to refuse: why shouldn't a few, key facilitators from a community get paid? You start a response, people get involved, they give up time and resources to respond: shouldn't someone be rewarded for that? The issue – like most issues connected to AIDS – lay in motivation or 'the heart', and money was perceived as changing the motivation.

Joseph's motivation was not in doubt: he had done this work for no financial reward for ten years; it seemed only fair he get something now, when he had a wife and children to support. The difficulty was that the regional response was not predicated on there being money, but on the community finding ways to generate the money themselves and building a response out of that. It was born out of a philosophy that people have an innate capacity to do this and that sometimes all it took was someone to help it happen.

In the early 1990s, the Africa Facilitation Team had visited many parts of Uganda and stimulated community responses focused on HIV and based on 'IGA' (Income Generating Activity): simple, twenty dollar catalytic efforts that in turn stimulated a lot of responses in communities through home care and community counselling. The result of the income generation within the community – just like the widows in Kithituni with Miriam the Cow and the jewelry making women in Makindu – was that they were then able to support the orphans themselves; a few at first, but slowly building to a point where a community, a series of communities, became capable of supporting orphans themselves, eventually on a scale that would have defeated far more affluent places. This is what we saw happening here in Kisekele. It was fantastic to behold a thousand orphans taken in by their own neighbours rather that being abandoned to the vagaries of an institution. But maybe only in Africa could the inherent community strengths have allowed such a thing.

It also takes faith to say no to money. The Salvation Army's regional response team had been operating on the long term, sustainable ideal that it was care, not money that leads to change. It was the antithesis of the Western, can-do, quick-fix, goal-orientated mentality; a mindset that is impatient, even intolerant of slow, unseen changes. PEPFAR was a welcome Western government intervention but while the money was needed, the approach did not really allow for a community voice. The interventionist approach – where huge dollops of money get thrown at a problem – tended to come with an attendant set of problems: the energy taken for organisation – project writing, documenting, human resource development – detracted from the expansion of local responses and lead to weariness, overwork and a preoccupation with systems and structures. 'Doing good' distilled to bureaucracy.

On our way to a 'community conversation' we stopped to pick up the Salvation Army district officer in Bumbo: Major Augustus Webaale. I had met him at the gathering of a thousand orphans but not had time to speak with him at length. He was a lovely looking man, statuesque and calm, like Nelson Mandela in mien and character. We were invited into his home, a simple but quietly elegant house. On the walls there were some framed photographs, including one of Augustus and his wife, dressed in full uniform, and standing in front of a red brick house under the kind of sky you only get in England.

He saw me looking and was quick to explain:

'Nottingham.' He said.

Nottingham was the birth place of William Booth. Augustus then produced a photograph album of a visit he and his wife had made to England a few years ago. The pictures were artless and prosaic: he and his wife outside the officer training centre in Sydenham; he and his wife and a group of fellow cadets by a statue of William Booth preaching in Mile End Road, London; he and his wife at the bus stand on their way to Heathrow Airport. As I looked I realised that I had seen these photos before, in India. Only the people in the photos were different. Major Randive and his wife had done the same visit (as honoured and promising overseas officers) and on that visit they had also done the essential Salvation Army pilgrimage and posed for photos at the site of their founder's birth place.

How grim and grey England looked in those pictures; how unlovely compared to this lush and spectacularly arranged stretch of Uganda. And yet, I could tell that Major Augustus had been greatly moved by his visit to England and that through us he was momentarily transported back to a time of feeling especially honoured. Maybe he had glimpsed something there that had given him a greater sense of his mission here. Britain, for him, was a place from which good things came. For me, every passing mile we travelled in the messy boot-prints of my country's colonial past undermined this greatness, but I didn't have the heart to disabuse my host of his idealised image of England, so I kept quiet.

Joseph and the Major accompanied us to something called a community conversation in the heart of N'mecha Corp. Community conversations are, as the name suggests, events at which all the people in an area come together and talk. In recent years, HIV/AIDS had been a forceful catalyst for bringing people together in this way. It has forced them to talk about some very difficult things; things traditionally left unsaid. HIV/AIDS has a habit of holding up a mirror and magnifier at a community and saying 'Look, this is what you are really like; what are you going to do about it?' Much as the Church throughout Africa has had its robes ruffled by a disease that goes to the heart of our humanity, so tribal communities – where essential decisions were usually taken by a chief or headman – had found their usual way of doing things completely challenged.

The community conversation was a natural social response and some believe it is the place where real change – or at least the desire for real change – is best expressed. For that reason, all kinds of organisations, from the Salvation Army to the United Nations have put time and resources into encouraging these events. The intention was to draw on the natural organic power of conversation, inherent in most indigenous communities, surround it with inspired facilitators, and get everyone in the village – everyone – talking about subjects that have always been taboo.

On the way to the meeting, Joseph told me that polygamy* had been, and still was, a major cause of the spread of HIV/AIDS in this eastern region of Uganda. But because it was traditional – cultural – the practice remained unchallenged. But in the last few years, through community conversations, people had voiced their own doubts about the wisdom of multiple unions; not because of some newfound doctrinal conviction but because HIV/AIDS had killed a lot of people through it. The same thing had happened with the practice of 'cleansing the widows' (a ritual which involved a new widow sleeping with the brothers of her deceased husband at the funeral itself in an effort to cleanse her of the spirit of death); female circumcision had also been rejected: a result of people talking about it. The urgency of AIDS gave people a greater boldness in saying things they'd never said before and this was leading to changes in behaviour and practice that had been in their culture for years.

The community conversation took place in a building in a field in Butselitsi. We could only drive so close before we had to park up and walk the rest of the way – about a mile – through a landscape that was richly soiled and green compared to the dry fields of Kithituni; and where the mud and straw homes were like a model village built for the 'Africa' section of an Expo. Once again, it was always hard to reconcile the peaceful allure of an African landscape with the strife that was going on within it.

This 'conversation' had not been specially arranged for our benefit; it was taking place anyway, as it did every week at the same venue. Attendance wasn't mandatory, but few would miss out on getting a chance to say something. By the time we arrived

* It is thought by many in the field, including Ian Campbell, that safe polygamy is better than unsafe promiscuity.

the building was as full as it could be: maybe 150 people: children, teenagers, men and women and the elderly. It really was the community gathered.

The topics for today's discussion had been written up on an A2 flipchart presenter. It was not going to be a trivial chit-chat. First up: the lack of support given to orphans and vulnerable children; that was to be followed by 'community awareness of HIV/AIDS'; the stigmatisation of the infected was next; then 'the need for counselling and guidance of orphans'; we'd finish with the issue of unfaithful partners; over-drinking and, if there was time, 'how poverty affected their community'.

The first people to speak were, appropriately enough, a group of orphans. One girl described her life: losing both her parents in the same year and then going to live with her aunt and uncle. She was remarkably candid about how difficult this was for her – and for her new parents, who were there in the hut with her. Her new parents had their own children; they naturally favoured their own kith and kin. She felt angry. Angry with her dead parents for dying; and angry with her new parents for not loving her as much as her old parents did. Life was hard and she had thought about ending it. The only thing that gave her hope was the Kids Club and being with other orphans who understood what it was like to lose your mother and father.

A young man who was chairing the conversation thought it time to highlight some of the topics that this story had raised. He announced that we would witness a mini roleplay entitled: 'How to Love An Orphan.'

A man and a child then enacted a scene in which an orphan was being adopted by new parents. The child – I don't know if he was an actual orphan – mimicked losing his parents; the man put an arm around him and led him to the imagined home; there the orphan was happy for a while (smiles); then the sad face returned: the other children, the real children, were getting all the privileges. The child walked away and faced the wall.

The chairman asked the gathering: How should we treat this child? He asked for someone to demonstrate. A man came forward and began to speak to the child.

'My brother's son, I love you, despite the fact that your father is dead, I am going to take care of you. But tomorrow you must get up and go to school to be a good citizen.'

We then heard from a mother of four who had taken on her dead sister's children. 'Since their parents passed away it is difficult' she said. 'They are not your own children. Church helps with food and materials. But it is a tug of war. I don't have much money.' The adoption, she went on, had also taken its toll on her marriage: her husband, who liked to drink beer, could not make enough money to support them all; she had only managed to survive because of some help from the Church; but there was only so much to go around.

As the woman spoke there was a swell of knowing '*Mmmm*'s. Most of the women could relate to what she was saying. Some women raised their voices as she told her story and, emboldened by it, echoed her words: 'Yes, these men and their beer!' This encouraged the woman to go further in her dispatch from the front line of her daily life. She said: 'It is impossible for the woman to do all of these things: to raise children, to cook, to cultivate the *shambas*, and then have the man come back from drinking beer all day and bring nothing. They act like they are the big boss. And they do nothing. They sleep around. Have other women. They expect it. They think they can because their fathers did this. This has to change!' By now there was a huge swell of assent; and the laughter and clapping was not just from the women.

It can take a generation to show a willingness to even address a subject like gender equality or male promiscuity and here, in a single hour, we seemed to have got to the essence of the problem that had plagued every country we'd been to so far. The problem of male fidelity and sobriety had an affect on pretty much every sphere of life; it was a conduit for AIDS, family break-up, abuse of women, and poverty; and part of it connected with a thing that was hard for people – indigenous and outsiders – to confront: cultural practice.

Stephen Lewis, a former ambassador to the UN and a passionate and outspoken advocate of the community conversation had little truck for pussy-footing around something traditionally felt politically incorrect to even discuss changing. He said 'Tackling culture head on – and deliberately – can cause huge transformation quickly. This dismal belief that it will take aeons stops us from doing what must be done and keeps us locked into the morbid belief that culture is a force we will not/cannot/may not change. There are only two things that have to change and change fast – it's the massive violence against women and children across the world; and the role of culture in protecting/encouraging violence and reducing HIV transmission. No culture is more sacred than life.'

The meeting ended with another song from a group of orphans. They were a little nervous and made a false start before the leader bade them begin again and they sang a song that stayed in our heads long after we'd left the fields of Butselitsi.

A week before – in the field of a thousand orphans – we'd heard a song: *you steal away my mother; you steal away my father*. In that song the 'you' was the anthropomorphised demon plague AIDS; it was this plague that was to blame for making them orphans; but in this song the children sang '*Ewe mama, ewe papa*' – 'Why mother, why father – were you not careful? Why did you not think of us or yourselves.'

The dead were not there to give an answer but the implication was stark and uncompromising. The children were implying that their own parents had let them down because they had done something without considering the consequences for themselves or their children. It was sometimes easy to forget in all the argument that many men and women had died from AIDS not because they didn't have a condom, enough money or enough ARVs but because they took a chance on sleeping with someone other than their spouse. Both the funerals I had attended in Kithituni were for men who had acquired the disease in this way. But maybe only the orphans of dead parents have the moral authority to question the actions that had left them bereft. When children are asking the older generation the question, 'Is it okay to sleep around?' then change is already happening.

That week, Gabriel and Agnes asked us if we could adopt an orphan. They had asked us the same question after visiting the drop-off centre for children of sex-workers in Mumbai and they would ask the question again in Soweto and – towards the end of the journey – in Henan province, China. Given the amount of abandoned children they encountered, shook hands with and played with and the circumstances these children were living in compared to their own, it was a reasonable question. It was manifestly obvious to them that there were more than enough children needing help and that we had the capacity to do something about it.

Nicola and I had talked about this, but only in abstract terms. I suspected that there would be a moment when we were tempted to do it and in a village, near Kisekele, on our last day in the district, we had that moment. We were on a home visit and I had sat in a kitchen with an orphan on my knee for several minutes listening to his adoptive mother tell me that it was sometimes very hard to look after other people's children, even if they were related to you. It was hard to love them as your own and they often came with emotional and psychological problems. She herself had taken on four orphans on top of the four children of her own. The boy was called David and he was beautiful and he seemed well and cheerful. 'What if we did?' flashed through my mind; but it was still only a thought. Our weeks there had cured us of any ideas we might have had about adoption. The response there demonstrated, fantastically, the capacity for communities to take upon themselves the burden of supporting their own orphans. They recognised what we already suspected: that orphans fared better, socially and emotionally, if they were able to remain part of the community. Despite the difficulty of raising extra children in these places, everyone agreed that it was still best for the orphans to be with their own people and for their own people to take them in.

The four of us took a car from Mbale in Uganda to the Kenyan border where we were picked up by a cousin of our driver and taken on to the city of Kisumu on the shores of Lake Victoria. Our driver was a tall, handsome man called Ahmed. Ahmed was a Muslim and on the way to Kisumu we got into a discussion about Islam and Christianity. Ahmed was intelligent and keen and he soon began to proselytise. At first he talked about the order and success that Islam brought to its adherents. How in Kenya, the Muslim community was far more successful in business than the non-Muslim. For him, Islam brought harmony through law, through offering clear guidelines as to how to live.

Once he knew we were Christian he switched his tack from describing Islam's merits; to pointing out Christianity's shortcomings. They were theological rather than practical objections and they centred on the impossibility – the blasphemy in fact – of God becoming man. This led to a lively but good-humoured discussion about the person of Jesus – who he was, what he said, what he did, what his followers should do – before ending on the issue of whether religion and freedom were compatible. He believed people needed rules and the poor state of Kenya and of Africa showed what happened when people didn't have guidelines. Particularly when it came to marriage and sex. He reserved his strongest words of disapproval for the tribal way of life, here in Kenya and in Africa generally. He said that HIV/AIDS was a big problem because of this way of life.

'Do you mean polygamy?' I asked him.

He paused. 'Not just that. But all kinds of things.'

'Does Islam do anything to help people infected with HIV/ AIDS?'

'The Koran teaches us to show mercy to the sick. And we have *zakat*. Giving alms to the poor. We all do this.'

'But do you do it yourself, or do you give the money to the mosque and they distribute the money?'

'The mosque distributes the money.'

'And if you meet someone who has HIV/AIDS what do you say to them? How can you help them?

'We have many programmes to help these people.'

'But do you go to them; or do they come to you?'

'They come.'

'But do they have to be Muslims?'

'I think so.'

We drove on for a while in silence before I asked him how many wives he had.

He had two.

I had to ask: 'Which one is your favourite? You must prefer one to the other.'

He smiled and shook his head.

'This is a real problem for me,' he said. 'My first wife does not like my second wife. She wants to kill her!'

He explained how since taking a second wife (his faith permitted four wives) his first wife had turned against him. It was reaching the stage where he might have to divorce her. He would look after her of course, his faith had strict guidelines about settlements for divorced wives; but it was making life difficult.

'Do you think we were made to have more than one wife?' I asked him.

'It is not for every man to do this,' he said. 'I used to think that I would have four wives, as the law permits, but now I am thinking I will have one. It is better to love one. It is easier to be faithful when you love your wife.'

Intermission

'Too far for you to see
The fluke and the foot-rot and the fat maggot'
– R.S. Thomas

A week after standing in 'the field of a thousand orphans', I was standing in the middle of the Serengeti Plain, a hundred miles from the nearest town, in a hot shower, in a luxury, centrally heated tent, furnished with four poster beds and Egyptian cotton sheets, after having had a meal of smoked salmon, roast beef, sorbet and a bottle of Cabernet Sauvignon, having spent the day on the back of a topless Toyota Land Cruiser looking at elephant, lion and cheetah, feeling a confusion of emotion; an uneasy tossed salad of gratitude, awe and embarrassment at what man is capable of achieving if he really wants something and how awry his priorities can get. To come across this superlative luxury in a country that can't even tarmac its main roads; or give its children free secondary education; or supply and distribute water to the bulk of its population is a kind of disgrace for which it's hard to know who to blame.

But how quick we were to convince ourselves that we deserved it and in the process forget the way most people actually have to live. The safari was an escape: from the road; from suffering; from AIDS; from Church. From bad food; from pit latrines; from endless handshakes and interviews; an escape from 'doing good'. It was also reward for the children, for the hard miles they'd done with little respite and few complaints. And it was indeed, a holiday unlike any other. Few things can touch the sight of a bull elephant at sunset or a giraffe running, or the thrill of danger at being within ten feet of an animal that can kill you; but I could never quite lose the niggling feeling that this pleasure was at someone else's expense or forget the people we'd met who, despite living in this country, had never seen such things. I thought of Big Agnes back in Kithituni. She was nearly seventy years old and she had never seen the *simba*.

We were allocated a game driver for the duration of our stay and, but for one game drive, we had him all to ourselves. His name was Rashid. He was an Asian Kenyan and he had been a game-driver for five years. It was a job and it was a prized job but the cost to him was being apart from his wife and son for three months in every six.

For the first day – spurred on by our enthusiasm and excitement at being in the bush – he talked about how great his job was. On the second day he said seeing my children reminded him of the children he was not with. He had two, like me, and his boy in particular missed his father. On the last day, he confessed that he would give up this job if he could to be with his wife and children, but he could not afford to do this because he supported his entire extended family off the back of his wages. He was not alone in this. Most of the staff that worked at the lodge endured long separations. One of the receptionists at the lodge told me that she had left her three-month-old baby with her mother for three months rather than give up her job. When it came down to it, these relatively well-paid, job-secure Kenyans were open to the same fragmentation of family, the same costs of dislocation, trials of separation and temptations faced by the truck drivers we had met in Sultan Hamud off the Mombasa Road.

Not that many people in the lodge had any idea about this. And why would they? The safari was a bubble into which anaesthetised, inoculated tourists landed and departed without ever once getting a sense of the wildlife – the raw struggle going on beyond the electric fence. Part of me envied those who flew in (through no fault of their own) to Nairobi, checked into the Hilton, checked onto a propeller plane that flew them to the Masai Mara, then, three days later on to the Indian Ocean beaches beyond Mombasa before returning them, tanned and replete to their Nairobi hotel and flight home. It must be easy to believe that Africa is a great place where the problems are not quite as bad as they say when this is the extent of your engagement with it. It must be easier to enjoy the 'journey of a lifetime' that the safari is said to be, when you are ignorant of or have been sheltered from seeing what is out there.

But it wasn't just the rift valley of economic difference that made it hard to fully enjoy the experience. The posters said 'Experience the Real Africa' but the safari had become to Africa what the Wild West was to America: an ersatz cultural-historical experience in which you tracked animals and had immaculate Masai dance for you while you drank Lavazza coffee after your four-course meal. It reminded us that too much of what we knew about this country – this continent – had come to us via the besotted views of colonials who seemed to have a mystical reverence for 'their Africa'. *Out Of Africa, Born Free, Gorillas in the Mist*. Blixen, Adamson, Fossey – they all seemed to be people who loved Africa – its land and its animals – before they loved its people. As Dervla Murphy wrote in the *Ukimwe Road*: '...their powerful accounts had hypnotised us into forgetting the realities behind the long grass – the destruction of delicately balanced relationships between land and people, herds and people, wildlife and people – people and people.' These love affairs with Africa's physical environment and wildlife almost stopped people from engaging with its people at all and instead encouraged them to keep their gazes fixed on the view.

The Boy in the Photograph

10th December, 2004

Dear Mrs Brook.

How are you? I am fine and every-body at home is fine.

I have closed school. I was position number twenty-seven. I was happy to close school.

I will help my mother to look after my younger sister Muthoni.

I will be playing with my twin brother Machoyia and my friend Ben football.

I love writing and recording.

Thank you very much for becoming my friend.

I pray for you everyday. Pray for me and my family.

Greet Gabriel and Agnes.

Patrick Nduati.

This was the first letter we received from a boy called Patrick Nduati who we had sponsored though an organisation called Compassion, two years before we made this journey. I can't recall exactly why we decided to sponsor a child (it was before we knew anything about our future assignment) but I think it was the eve of the Make Poverty History campaign and questions such as 'What can we do?' were in the ether and filtering through to our consciences. By the time Nicola saw the leaflet we were already looking for a way to make some kind of connection. Sponsoring a child seemed like a small but tangible step towards doing something about 'the things we saw on the news'.

Our children were captivated at the idea of having 'a brother' in Africa and took to writing and exchanging photographs with Patrick. From Patrick's pencil written letters and photographs we tried to piece together a picture of his life. The boy in the photograph was one year younger than my son; he had a direct and serious countenance and looked to be wearing his 'Sunday best'. He seemed to come from a family of faith because his letters were filled with promises of prayer and praise. He lived with his mother, two brothers and sister, near Kenya's 'third' city, Nakuru – famous for its saline lake and a congregation of a million flamingos – in the hills of Engashura, in a house he seemed to spend a lot of time helping his mother clean. His mother worked as a farm labourer when she could and earned the equivalent of fifteen pounds per month, an amount that left little for the luxuries of schooling or new clothes. Patrick's father was alive but did not live with the family. This last piece of information wasn't something Patrick disclosed; it was there in the little file we were given about him. It didn't say why the father wasn't there but the inference was that Patrick and his family needed support because of his absence. For two years we exchanged letters with Patrick and paid our eighteen pounds a month to Compassion – money that provided him with spiritual, academic and vocational support and (we would later see with our own eyes) his entire family with a semblance of a living. When we learned that we would be making the journey and that Kenya was to be a key destination, we made a commitment to visit him. We would go to the lake of a million flamingos and then see the boy in the photograph for real.

The letter from Compassion, regarding the arrangement for our visit, expressed great excitement at our coming to see Patrick. Few sponsors got the opportunity to actually meet the child they sponsor and a visit was, they said, a powerful demonstration of 'how much you care'. We were glad to have this time to move the relationship on from words on paper to deeds in flesh, but we were slightly apprehensive as we drove to meet Patrick with the two representatives from Compassion. We were hoping this visit would be more than benevolent donor meets needy recipient.

Our children were free from such tortured speculation. They were rightly curious and abuzz about meeting Patrick; for a week they had talked about what gift they were going to give him. Gabriel had bought a thorn-proof football and decided to give his fake replica Manchester United shirt that he'd bought from the market in Aizawl, Mizoram. Given that most young men in football-crazy Africa seemed to support one of the four leading English Premiership football teams, there was a one in four chance of Patrick being a Manchester United supporter.

Patrick and his mother were waiting for us at his local church community centre, along with the church minister and the local Compassion representatives. If those first few moments were stiff and awkward for us; they must have been strange for Patrick and his mother. The language barrier made the initial interaction feel leaden and 'a bit UN'. The translator translated our careful-to-be-sensitive questions and took little time translating Patrick's short, shy answers. If Patrick was moved but slightly bewildered by us, his mother was emotional and her emotion expressed itself in a tearful speech of thanks to us for coming and for helping support Patrick – and the family. She gave an impressively detailed account of what the eighteen pounds a month had enabled her to do for him. We were then shown Patrick's schoolwork, recording his spiritual as well as academic progress. It was good to see his work but hard to fully engage; we made interested noises – and we were interested – but I didn't feel I had any right to assess the boy's work; it felt like a hastily arranged parent's evening at a school for one.

The mood lightened once we got out to Patrick's home, which was high up on the hills of Engashura Farm, away from the main roads and the city. His home was like a thousand other homes we'd seen: about the size of a single garage, dirt floor, mud walls and corrugated tin roof. Another hut opposite served as a home for his sister and her husband. There was a cluster of curious neighbours around the huts and a lot of laughing at and with us as we made our way inside for a cup of tea.

It was dark inside the home; something that always bothered us, being people from the Northern Hemisphere who spent more time in than out. We sat in a circle on stools, smiled at each other and drank tea. The walls were bare but for some public health posters illustrating the importance of drinking and using clean water. One of the posters showed how to build a pit latrine. The only other decorative things were the homemade coverlets on the chairs and the cross weave tablecloth. When we had tried to imagine Patrick's house from his letters, we had conjured a more ideal house: less dark, handcrafted furniture; simple but somehow more 'idyllically African' than this.

The children broke the ice by presenting Patrick with his Manchester United shirt. He immediately got up and pulled it on over his own shirt. His twin brother pulled at the shirt and laughed at his brother who smiled for the first time. Gabriel then gave Patrick a football that his twin brother took for himself. If we were worried at all this attention – and support – being lavished on one boy, we needn't have been. Even if you wanted your money to go to one person, the African way of life simply wouldn't have allowed it: they are too community minded; they will spread the resources according to the need and – particularly if the mother is the purser – more fairly than any bank or NGO could contrive. It was good to see how well and how far the money went, but salutary seeing how much difference such a relatively small amount to us made to them.

The women cooked on a stove outside: *japatis* were being rolled and fried and a feast being prepared. Patrick's mother was keen to show us her gratitude. The young woman helping with the cooking was – his mother told us – one of Patrick's sisters from a previous marriage. Patrick's mother said that she had nine children in total. I wanted to ask what happened to the first husband but it didn't seem right to ask. I also wanted to know where Patrick's father was now (we knew he was alive) but it didn't seem right to ask either. What was it that had led these fathers to leave the home: economics? Lust? Beer? Discovering their HIV status? Or could they simply not face the burden of being a father? Maybe it was the same answer for both her ex-husbands.

Patrick wanted us to see his bedroom so we all trooped in, one at a time, to see it: a small, dark room with one wooden bed that Patrick shared with his twin brother. The bed was covered with a homemade quilted blanket and clothes hung above the bed in the fashion of an open wardrobe. A satchel hung on a hook on the cracked wall. Everything we could see was everything he owned.

The women called us back to eat and I was asked to say a grace. I spoke it slowly to allow the man from Compassion to translate. I started with a thanks for the food but soon moved on to thanks for Patrick, and then on to his mother, his brother and sisters and the volunteers from Compassion and then the community. It was a proper African grace, missing no opportunity or object to be grateful for and ending – mindful of absent fathers – with thanks to the Father of all. Why does saying grace come easier in places where there is materially less to thank God for?

We ate a wonderful meal. The beans were the best beans we'd had in Africa and the chicken pieces – unlike the chicken we ate in Kithituni – actually had meat on. We mopped up the juice with sweet, white bread and clinked our soda bottles together in a sequence of toasts. Eating together changed the dynamic of the day. Gone was the donor-recipient apprehension; we were all equals now – brothers and sisters sharing a meal – and we were the ones being given to. The conversation eased, we passed beyond the formal and began to laugh and joke and enjoy the fact that we were two different families made one for a few, fleeting hours.

'Write My Name Somewhere'

We had been away for two months. We had travelled across the Indian Ocean, across the Indian sub-continent, back to Africa and into its heartland. It was a mark of how quick and deep our time in Kithituni had been in that first month that through all our wanderings we considered it to be our emotional and spiritual base camp. At certain low points on our journey (induced by minor ailments, travel fatigue or just plain world weariness) we had got homesick and thought of 'normal life' back in London and missed it; but by the time we returned to Kithituni it felt like coming home.

We came back to a rain-soaked landscape and a hope-soaked people. The red dust road from Sultan Hamud had become an ochre mud track and there were now two bubbling rivers to negotiate before reaching April's house. The *matatus* and trucks formed a reluctant snake at the first of these and Mark, spotting a gap and trusting to the car's suspension, drove on through, sluicing and careening like a rally car. This rain (coinciding with our return) was what the people had been waiting for; not the phoney rains we'd had just before we'd left for Rwanda, but these riverbed-filling, truck-stopping rains that got people planting and things growing.

We had come back to a changed topography: what had once been yellow was now green, what had been blue was now grey, and what had been red was now brown. The landscape was luminous with a liquid sheen and the people were shining too, from sweat. Languid waiting had turned to frantic digging. On both sides of the road people were at their *shambas* hoeing, raking, ploughing and planting. It looked frenetic and random, like the 'drop-everything' grabbed opportunity that it was.

Mark explained: 'People have to plant while they can. Just in case this is it. The danger now is that the rains will be too strong and wash everything away.' Everyone we knew – old, young, man, woman – seemed to be busy tending their *shamba*: George the Baptist, Major James, Joseph and Georgie-Porgie; Agnes, Abednego, even Thomas the Goatherd.

It was an auspicious time to come back: by association we were a blessing. 'When "The Rhidians" come, the rain comes. It rained a little last time you came. And now it rains again – only this it is the real rains.' Mark said. 'They will be calling you Wamboa and Mumbua – Mr and Mrs Rain.'

There was no better thing to be known for in these parts.

The next morning I walked into the town and met Mark's brother, (Martin's father) Jacob, on the road. It was now impossible to ride a bicycle because of the mud so I pushed it and talked to my neighbour. I wanted to know what was going on in his world; he wanted to know what was going on in the world out there. Us coming back was a good thing; but the going away and the distance we had gone was unsettling to him. He had not travelled much, even by the standards of the locals; but he was curious to know things:

'Do they have an AIDS problem in India?'

'Do they have much poverty in India?'

'Do you like Kithituni better than these other places you have seen?'

Yes. Yes. And Yes.

He was relieved at all three of my answers. The fact of there being poverty in another country – even a country as seemingly great as India – reassured him. The fact that we had been to these places – the great cities of Mumbai and Calcutta and Kenya's neighbouring countries – and still preferred his hometown gladdened him. His was a fragile pride: he was intelligent and aware enough to know that he lived in a poor place; but he could see that it was a place that sophisticated, well-travelled *muzungus* seemed hugely happy to get back to. The more I said how good it was to be 'home' the more avuncular he became: 'Have you lost weight? You look a bit thin,' he said. The implication being: a few weeks back here will see you right.

'Everybody missed you very much,' he said. 'Yes. Very much.' And I knew that he was speaking for himself when he said this.

That first month, I had tried to convey something of the shock, wonder and enigma of Kithituni through rushed emails sent from the goat-powered internet in Henry's grain store. Email had been our main means of communication with friends and family back home. It leant itself well to the unmitigated, first flush of encounter. I wanted to give people a flavour, without filtering out; but a part of me was conscious of making more of something than was actually there. Is this as wonderful, as heightened, as I am saying? Would others see it this way? What if some people came and experienced it, too? Would they see it the way I had described it? Would they accuse me of seeing what I wanted to see?

When we learned that our friends from home – Adam and Jules – were going to come and see us I had that mixed feeling of excitement at seeing people we knew well and the possessive insecurity that comes of sharing something that has become precious. Kithituni had become 'our' place; it was one thing sharing a place with people through words and virtual sensation; but to share it physically, to let others come and see it – even close friends – was to test the cosy assumptions we'd made and risk having our own views challenged.

Our friends were actually doing the very thing that I had challenged them to do: namely, the next time you take a safari try and engage with what is going on in the rest of the country. They only had three days with us, but they wanted to see, taste and smell as much of what we'd talked and written about as they could. It wasn't going to be full engagement, but it was a start. We set them up with a visit to the Kibera – straight off the back of their safari in the Masai Mara – and then a two day 'immersion' in the community HIV/AIDS response: with a visit to the women's 'banana group' and a home visit to see Pascal – Onesmus's uncle – and Martha who I had visited with the team that first month in Kithituni.

The locals in the town were excited to hear that friends of 'The Rhidians' were coming from London to see Kithituni.

The evening they arrived we cooked as fine a meal as was possible for us to cook using the remainder of supplies from Nairobi and some goat meat we had bought at market. Goat meat is a tough, slightly gamey meat and full of flavour. Adam – who liked good wine – had bought half a mixed case of staggeringly fine vintage at Heathrow.

Outside in-flight beer, we had adopted a teetotal policy in keeping with our adopted Salvation Army sensibilities. Buying wine in Kithituni was out of the question anyway; and the culture of drinking was frowned upon in most African rural areas, starkly dividing into those who drink (madmen, bad-men, wasters and thieves) and those who don't (the hard working, the sensible and the sane). There didn't seem to be a middle ground.

But we came from that middle ground and our friends had come a long way to see us and there was no way that roast goat wasn't going to be washed down with that Claret. And even though we didn't have a fridge to cool it, the Chablis would be drunk lukewarm under the stars.

How good and powerful it was to taste in that wine something of the complexity and beauty and culture of the world we came from and hear in the familiar rhythms and reference points of our friends' conversation something of ourselves that we'd forgotten about on the journey. We had not missed such things because we had been so immersed in a new and challenging way of life; but to be with people who spoke the same language, made us realise how little we'd actually talked in the way that we might have done had we been back in England. It was like using a muscle we hadn't used for months and it was helpful to be able to process something of what we had seen on the journey so far with people who – like us – were used to a more comfortable way of being.

A few weeks later – after our friends had gone – Jacob and Margaret came to dinner with us and noticed the wine bottles: which we were now using as candle-holders. When Jacob saw them he looked amazed and intrigued.

'You had wine?'

'Yes'

'Really? What is it like?'

'It's pretty good.'

'I cannot imagine drinking it.'

'Maybe when you come to London, you will try some.'

'I should very much like to go to London,' he said. 'But not to drink wine.'

We took Adam and Jules on a home visit with the team to see Pascal and Martha, the two people – both HIV positive – who I had visited in that first action-packed week when the team wanted to show me everything they could. I remembered my own response to that visit: the awe I felt at people's willingness to spend a whole day visiting one or two sick people and the exasperation at seeing they had nothing but themselves to take. The tightrope walk between sadness and disappointment, hope and victory with faith the balancing pole that kept them up. I wondered if my friends would see what I thought I had seen.

On the way to *rendez-vous*ing with the team at Agnes's café we met Jonathan in the grain house. And Big Agnes in the market. And Henry at the money counter. And Sylvester on the road. And Mrs Major outside the Onion Lady's stall. People had heard that there were visitors and visitors needed to be seen, shaken and patted properly. We then decamped to Agnes's to meet with the team. The sudden need to tend *shambas* meant some people were late or not able to come. Joseph had okra to deliver; Georgie-Porgie had a river in full flow to cross now and that added an hour to his journey. We waited until everyone had arrived (it was never known how many would show – it was a mystical and organic process). Once everyone was there who we thought would be there, Onesmus outlined the purpose of our visit, Johnnie Boy prayed for the visit, we sank our sodas, and set off.

It was hot and humid by the time we traipsed up the hillside to see Pascal and it was not yet ten o'clock. We numbered fifteen in all: fifteen people to spend six hours visiting two people. Was this – as I had fervently come to believe – the economics of love; or the economics of inefficiency? I wanted to believe that it was the former and I wanted my friends to see it too; for them to get beyond the Western system for measuring success. It was odd, this protectiveness of mine because this work was a great thing and a thing that needed to be seen to be appreciated. It was as if I'd discovered a secret that by its very hidden, fragile nature might not stand up to scrutiny.

Pascal had deteriorated in the three months since our last visit. Then he had been standing upright; now he sat sunken in a chair in a suit jacket and baseball cap, the belt around his trousers as tight as it could go. He was cadaverous, his cheekbones jutting and his white teeth seemingly too big for his mouth; he smiled beautifully for us by way of greeting but he did not seem to have the muscles to sustain it. We asked him how he was and he told us that he was not doing too well. The doctors weren't sure why he was not responding to the treatment. He said his T cell count was below 100 and that he needed to get to the hospital (fifty miles away) to get some more ARVs.

Pascal was listless and his concentration wandering but he seemed determined to stay with us and give an answer to every question, even if it took him a while to formulate his thoughts. Careful of his condition, we asked light, polite questions; questions asked as much from our own awkward feelings of how to be natural with a man who knew he was dying and who knew that we knew. What is your favourite animal (leopard)? What is your favourite colour (green)? When is your birthday (October – six months away)? What would you like for your birthday?

Pascal saw through it:

'Why do you ask me these questions? Let us talk about important things,' he said. 'You are a writer, yes? Then you must write the things that matter.'

I asked him how he caught the virus.

He said he used to live 'another kind of life' in Mombasa – and he thinks he caught it from his first wife.

Was his first wife still alive?

No.

What is the answer – to stop this pandemic?

He said it was up to us to tell the people about AIDS. To tell the children. Educate them. Teach them to live well and to live right. To be faithful. The Church can help, he said. These people here (the team) are helping. He said he was grateful to these visits from the team and that they had kept him alive, made his life worth living. There was a time, not so long ago, when he had lost his faith and stopped going to church. But these people had brought the church to him. They had given him faith and he was not afraid.

As he spoke, Pascal seemed to become more authoritative like a man dispensing the best of what wisdom he had been given before he was no longer around to pass it on.

Did he feel afraid?

Of death? No. He felt peaceful, despite his situation. He knew death was coming for him but the prospect did not frighten him. He said he had prayed and that he knew that God was going to take care of him. Pascal talked like a man with a longer view of things. Believing that God would take care of him – after death – was taking the long view.

At the end, maybe an hour later, after we had prayed with him and for him, he turned to me and asked:

'What are you going to do?'

'I am going to write about what I have seen,' I said. 'Tell people.'

He took my hand and held it with a gentle, prompting, urgent strength.

'Good,' he said. 'Will you do something for me?'

'Yes,' I said.

'Remember to write my name somewhere.'

Miracle in Machakos

'The real philanthropists in our society are those who work for less than they can live on'
— Jim Wallace

Jackson was the man responsible for designing and building April's house. He would show up from time to time to check on the men's progress. He was built like a heavyweight boxer, but he was gentle and precise and – we were soon to learn – modest. He was a man who had a vision for building things that lasted; there was a perfectionism about his work which no amount of poor circumstance or lack of resource was going to hinder.

Jackson lived about an hour north-west, near the city of Machakos and had initiated his own HIV/AIDS community response in his village. He had invited the team to visit and see what good things had occurred there. It was a chance do a bit of what the team called 'transference': to exchange ideas and learn from another community's experience. But it was to prove much more than that for us.

We went in a *matatu* that we'd hired for the day – the whole team – and on the road we got into a conversation about marriage and, in particular, the bride price. A bride price (also known as bride wealth) was the amount of money or property paid to the parents for the right to marry their daughter. It differed from the dowry, (which is paid to the groom) and to my mind it seemed prohibitive, even deleterious for a generation struggling economically and yet looking for (and having dire need of) faithful commitment. I had heard that the minimum bride price was two goats and was wondering whether I should give our goats – Larium and Malarone – to one of the young men as a leaving present. Both Joseph and Johnnie Boy had said, in an earlier conversation, that they would wait to get married – maybe until they were thirty – because they could not yet afford the bride price.

The tribal economic system – like that of ancient Europe's – was based on cattle (the word 'pecuniary' comes from the Latin, *pecus*, cattle). The cows are not necessarily there to eat, or milk; they were the clan's bank account. And cows – as Mary and the widows had explained to me – were very expensive (about one hundred pounds sterling per head).

I threw out the questions: should we equate love with economics? Wasn't it better to encourage marriage by lifting these hefty tariffs? Weren't the young – with all the natural temptations and in the light of HIV/AIDS – better off getting married sooner rather than later? A lively discussion bubbled up, with a fairly robust defence of the bride practice coming from Oral Robert. For him the bride price was about community and economic balance. After all, the bride price was, in market terms, compensatory; a payment made in exchange for the bride's family's loss of a daughter's labour – and fertility. What became clear as we talked was that the Christian concept of union and one flesh and the rites of marriage carried less weight (even among these believers) than the honouring of the bride price. Oral Roberts said as much to me when he admitted that some of the difficulty in his own marriage (he and his wife were no longer living together) stemmed from her parents not being happy about the bride price that he thought had been agreed. They still had claims over her and therefore his marriage. The fact they had got married in the Anglican Church didn't overrule that claim.

Agnes – my daughter – was sitting on my knee as we discussed this. She was all ears.

'So, Mr Rhidian, how much will the bride price be for your Agnes? Have you decided? ' Margaret asked me.

'Well, allowing for inflation over the next ten years, I'd say it has to be at least ten goats.' People laughed but my priceless daughter sitting on my knee wanted to know what I'd said.

'I was just saying how much you were worth.'

'How much?'

'Ten goats.'

'That's not very much.'

'No.'

Jackson's village was a few miles shy of Machakos, close to the main road and spread over land that didn't seem like a natural place for a village to be settled: it was on a slope, had little tree cover and no river. The land – we later learned – had been given to 61 families 'set free' thirty years ago by the owner of the land – a white Englishman whose own family had farmed here since the 1930s. This superficially generous act had a catch: there was no water on or near the land, rendering it almost impossible to cultivate. The 'freedom' the farm labourers had gained was emasculated by the inadequacy of their new situation.

Jackson came to greet us at the main road, with some men from his village including another man known as Mambua – Mr Rain. And we could see – coming up the track towards us – a group of women, all dressed in matching brown and green wraps, singing a joyful welcome song.

'Here come our wives,' Mambua said.

The noises of welcome and the smiling and laughter that came with them enveloped us all. The two communities met on the road and there were hugs and hand slaps all round. The wives had formed their own women's group in the community and the matching dresses were complemented by the men who all wore matching green, long sleeved button shirts. It was a simple visible expression of community solidarity and – like the HIV/AIDS response work in Kithituni – it transcended denominational and tribal affiliations. This community had really had to learn a new way of doing things in order to survive. And Jackson – it turned out – had been the architect of much we were about to see.

As we walked into the village, I could see that there were pathways and that the pathways were hemmed in by hedges that were trimmed and shaped. There was a pattern and order to the place. Someone (Jackson) had put thought into the design of the village. And then there were the houses themselves with their big, black water tanks attached to their sides – each tank filled from the actual reservoir constructed by the men from the village in order to solve their water problem. What was remarkable was that these tanks were paid for by neighbours pooling their resources and setting something aside each month. One by one they were purchasing tanks for people and they had now bought eighteen in five years.

Some ten years ago, tired and fed up with their situation, Jackson and two friends decided to start a group, pooling their resources together. It was like a banana group, except they tried to get everyone in the village involved. Out of the saved funds the village were able to send two of their own – one of them being Jackson – to college. Jackson went on to study architecture. Now he was repaying his community in a spectacular way: digging reservoirs, purchasing water tanks, designing a clean and connected environment in which to live.

What little these people had they shared. It was an organic welfare system: paying for medicine, ARVs, mosquito nets and giving support to the orphans and widows. It didn't seem possible – going on the small, mustard-seed amounts that people set aside – but it worked, producing great fruit.

After the presentation of a brown and green skirt to Nicola and a green long sleeve shirt to me, we huddled inside one of the houses to eat lunch. It had started to rain and the rain was heavy and noisy on the tin roof of the house. While waiting for our food, we discussed the country, the government, the claims of corruption in the news.

There were two young men in the room who were active in their local constituency. One of them said that over the years, the Kenyan people '...have learned to do things for themselves. They cannot rely on government. They have lost trust.' The sadness, for him, was that the young Kenyans didn't think politics had any answers to their problems. The youth, he said, did not know much about their rights. Knowing a little about your rights enabled you to be active, to get things done.

His friend spoke of Moi, the former President of Kenya for twenty years before Kibaki. Moi was a strong leader, but in the old, Big Boss style. When Kibaki had come to power one of his first acts was to provide free universal primary education, something that Moi had never managed to achieve. When I asked why Moi hadn't managed this, the man said that it was in Moi's interests to keep his people uneducated. That way they would never find out what they were missing, or how much better things could be.

I could see Joseph, George and Johnnie listening intently to this. They themselves were – relatively speaking – educated and well-informed young men, but men for who political involvement was a thing seemingly beyond reach. These two men from Machakos spoke eloquently and inspirationally about having an effect in the wider world; but it wasn't just youthful, radical zeal, it was practical: they had made the connection between what was happening in communities like this and what might happen throughout the country. They believed that a community could influence a country through the small acts of ordinary men and women rather than relying on the grand gestures and rhetoric of potentates.

As we were about to be served, Wamboa mentioned that in their community they had a group of people – many of them in their eighties – who remembered what it was like to live under and work for the white farmer before they came to settle here. They were actually all here now, eating lunch in the rondaval next door.

'Maybe you would like to meet them?'

Who would not want to meet such a group and ask them for their views about life, about what they had seen, about AIDS, about colonialism?

Nicola and I took our enamel bowls with us to the neighbouring rondaval and there, sitting on benches, waiting for their lunch to be served, were about twelve men and women, ranging in age from about 65 to 90. The women wore a multi-coloured mix of skirts and scarves; the men wore jackets and hats, their silver hair visible and striking against their dark skin. One or two had green-blue eyes and their skin was a lighter colour than the others, almost mixed race.

We sat with them and Jackson joined us to interpret.

I said that we were from England. That I was a writer trying to understand AIDS and other things. I said I was interested to know their thoughts about AIDS but also their feelings – their true feelings – about life before, during and after the white farmer. Knowing that they would be innately respectful and loath to criticise, I encouraged them to speak the truth, even if they had to say bad things about my country and thought I might not like what I was going to hear.

A younger lady in white headscarf and knitted wool cardigan spoke first. She said that AIDS was a new problem and that it was because there was no faithfulness any more. She said that people used to be much more faithful but that now people were not. They did not have one partner. I asked if in their day people really were more faithful and all of them – the men included – said yes. Another lady, much older, said that AIDS reminded her of a disease they used to have in the village years ago. At the time they believed it was a disease of incest. It produced similar symptoms and caused people to waste away just like AIDS. (I had heard this theory before, from one of the elderly widows in Kithituni).

'Was life better in those days?' I asked.

There was a rumble in the room.

'Under the farmer we had all our basic needs taken care of. If you were sick and needed medicine. We had food and we had water. But life is better now that we are free.'

I asked if he would explain what life was like then – working for the farmer – and even before the farmer (some of these people actually went back far enough to remember life before the relatively late grab of land in this part of Kenya).

One of the old men stood up to speak, taking his hat in his hands and acted as an unofficial spokesman for the group. He said that he had fought for the British in the Second World War – in Burma. He and many of the men from his village were recruited to do this. They were told that they were fighting for freedom and they believed this. But when the war for freedom had been won and they returned to Kenya he realised that they were not free at all. They had gone to the other side of the world to fight against people who had taken land from people who had themselves taken his land.

'For whose blood?' he asked me. 'For whose blood?'

He went on to explain that he was later imprisoned by the British for being part of the Mau Mau uprising in the 1950s. An estimated 150,000 Kenyans were held in British prison camps for up to seven years during what was known as the Kenya Emergency, a rebellion against colonial rule. The camps were justified, in British eyes, by the Mau Mau's butchering of 32 white settlers and African chiefs loyal to the crown. In Britain the Mau Mau were portrayed as representing the re-emergence of primitive bloodlust that the twin benefits of colonialisation – Christianity and civilisation – were intended to eradicate. But the British proved themselves as brutal as their enemies.

The spokesman went on: 'We were exploited and tortured for

what was rightly ours. No one has ever said sorry for that.'

I was beginning to feel that there was something missing from my education; an education gained at a school founded by a ruthless and exploitative mercantile company and continued at a University built on capital extracted from the cheap labour of colonial tobacco plantations. Somehow, they never told me about this. Can it be with all that knowledge they didn't know? Maybe they were too ashamed to.

It was not his intention to make us feel bad, but we did and Nicola was moved enough to offer some kind of vicarious apology – on behalf of our nation – for the sins our fathers had committed against them.

Then the spokesman said that they did not blame us. It was in the past. This sentiment was given a firm assent by all present in the room. Where did they get such restraint, such grace from?

'You are very forgiving,' I said.

And then he looked at me and said something extraordinary:

'You (the British) took away our dignity, our freedom, our culture, our time, our family life; but someone brought us the gospel and because of that we can forgive you.'

The Economics of Love

'When you leave we will have a feast. We will kill two goats.'

'Which two goats? Our two goats?'

'No, no, they are babies. You will need two big goats from the market.'

'What should we do with the goats we have?'

'Give them to some families who are very poor. The lady over there and the orphans next to us. If we swap your boy goat for a girl goat then you can give two girl goats away. That way they can make more goats and then they can pass on the girl goats to another family.'

Margaret gave us this sound advice with a sad reluctance.

'But I do not want to think about you leaving.'

Later that week – our last in Kithituni – my family, led by Big Agnes and Margaret, took Malarone and the girl goat swapped for Larium to a neighbouring family and a hamlet where several AIDS orphans were being looked after by some families who were barely managing to support themselves. The goats were presented on our behalf with the sweet, sombre ceremony that attends all transactions here – however small. Big Agnes said a prayer that sounded like a poem and was as long as a ballad. Whether it was for a glass of water or a goat given away Big Agnes knew how to bless a moment. I asked Margaret what she was saying.

'She is asking God to multiply this gift.'

And there it was, the economics of love: take the step of

giving some small thing; give it gladly and freely and in the full expectation of it becoming more than just the thing you can see.

That week, a *matatu* came to April's house to pick up some passengers going to Makindu. Onesmus was on board and, seated just behind the driver, slouching forward and leaning on his stick was his Uncle Pascal. In the last few weeks Pascal's condition had deteriorated. He wanted to be taken to the hospital: his wife – who was also sick – could no longer look after him. Onesmus had raised enough money from people in the community to take his Uncle Pascal to the Mbilikani hospital, on the Tanzanian border. This hospital was originally established to serve the nomadic communities and Pascal, being Kamba, had to do what other non-nomadic communities did and fake tribal affiliation to gain admission there.

To get him there, Onesmus had to buy two seats in a *matatu* that was going to Makindu. The driver then had to be paid an additional amount to drive the extra forty miles to Mbilikani and back with only two passengers. The cost of paying the *matatu* driver to take Pascal and Onesmus the extra distance from Makindu was about thirty pounds sterling. This was a ridiculous amount of money, but Onesmus had few options. This profligate and make-do ambulance service was the product of many factors: poor roads, bad transport, few hospitals and inadequate structures for drug distribution. The hospital was the nearest hospital dispensing free ARVs. In the past it had always been cheaper to take Pascal to an outlet offering free ARVs via an expensive journey than to buy them from the nearer hospital in Makindu. It was hard not to feel anger and frustration at a scene in which a young man had to find the equivalent of a month's salary, give up a day of his time to take a man who was perhaps now beyond saving to a hospital that was over two hours drive away.

But this wasn't about what we thought. It was time to say

goodbye to a man who was probably making his last journey. Pascal himself had asked to be taken to the hospital and the previous day he had asked Onesmus to fetch the Major to come and pray for him. He knew where he was going. He wasn't quibbling over logistics.

We leant into the *matatu*, one by one, and held his hand. He was focusing all his strength on simply trying to sit up but he managed to smile and his grip was strong. He said he felt fine and was not afraid. Someone said a prayer for Pascal and we said farewell. Just as the *matatu* conductor prepared to slide the door shut, Pascal lifted up his fingers and beckoned me toward him. His voice was barely audible so I leant over to listen closer.

'Remember what I told you,' he said.

Then the morning of the day of our leaving feast, Lelu came back from market with two large goats. We had invited nearly every person we'd made any connection with and estimated that maybe about a hundred people would show up. Margaret and Lelu did the maths and guessed that two big goats – padded out with *japatis* and rice – would suffice. The banana group would make the *japatis*, cook the rice and make the goat stew; Agnes's café would supply sodas and vegetables; and Lelu, Onesmus and Johnnie Boy would kill, skin and roast the goats. Being the host, I felt it was something I should do myself, but incompetence in such a matter wouldn't have been fair on the goats. And I wasn't up for the blood. I stood on the porch and watched from afar while my daughter Agnes went out and stood a few yards from Lelu while he lay each goat down and slit its throat, leaving the blood to spill on and stain the red earth.

It was good to have something to organise on that last day; it took our minds off the melancholy of departure. The centripetal pull of excitement at moving on to the next thing was always strong on this journey; but in Kithituni it was countered by the centrifugal force of friendships and connections holding us there.

That evening we made a bonfire from the wood that lay around the garden; we made long bench seats from the beams unused in the construction of April's house; we set out two crates of soda and the women cooked *japati* and chopped up the goat. We looked nervously at the sky and the clouds overhead, scudding across from the mountains, spitting rain.

People started to arrive as the light was fading. Everyone in the community we had come to know came, although the first to arrive were two old women I'd never seen before, who took their goat stew and sodas and immediately started tucking in. Then the ministers arrived. We had invited them all: Major Mutungwa from the Salvation Army, George the Baptist and his family, as well as the Anglican priest and the Assemblies of God preacher – Anthony Manges – who had sold me his tracts and papers from his correspondence course in Manchester.

Later, they would each give a short speech (what minister could resist a gathering?): the Major was gentle and sad, George passionate, hopeful and grateful; and at the end a surprising speech from Anthony (who we knew less well) who said that by having a party like this we'd reminded the community of how things used to be: all tribes, all denominations meeting to eat and talk and celebrate life.

April was called to speak. She had been with us since that morning and I had watched her talking with the women as they cooked, hovering in the background, modest and unassuming and yet central to everything. She gave thanks to the community for looking after and over us and reminded us all of what it was that brought us here. Then each member of the team – Johnnie, Nessy, Anton, Robert, Joseph – spoke of the good times we'd had tramping the red roads, visiting people and they enacted a song and dance that recalled the miles we'd walked. Margaret spoke beautifully of family and marriage and friendship.

Then Jonathan and Agnes stepped forward and Jonathan spoke in his direct and soulful way. Later, upon our return, when people asked me what was the most amazing thing we saw on the whole journey, I would always see the faces of these two. You could tell the moment you met them that they were a kind of natural wonder. In a culture decimated by a disease that ruined relationships, broken families, killed parents, separated mothers and fathers, they were a freak of nature – an anomaly – a couple who had been married for fifty years, had thirteen children (who at that time were all alive), who had not succumbed to disease, who had remained faithful to each other and who were at the heart of all that was good and fruitful in their community.

After the benedictions, we were presented with gifts, carved, sewn and woven; and our stay here was concluded as it had been overtured: with a prayer. We had been in Kithituni no longer than four months, but we were sent away like people who had lived there a lifetime.

A Short History of Care

'Never doubt that a small group of thoughtful,
committed people can change the world.
Indeed, it is the only thing that ever has.'
— Margaret Mead

We travelled a thousand miles south, to Zambia; from humid equatorial heat to the crisp winter of the Southern Hemisphere; following the great wave of AIDS south towards the epicentre of the pandemic, to another community where small things had made a big difference. To Chikankata, where the Salvation Army had built a Mission Hospital seventy years ago, naming the place after the local headman – Charlie Chikankata – who gave them a plot of land on which to build. This was the hospital where, twenty years ago, Dr Ian Campbell and others, including our accompaniment for this journey – Captain Sherry Pelletier – had helped pioneer the work that had shaped and challenged the orthodoxies of AIDS response.

There were not many people in the wards the day we arrived. Of the patients that were there, only two were in for AIDS related illnesses. The rest were mainly children, in for malaria or domestic burns received from indoor charcoal burner cooking accidents. The lack of AIDS related patients in the hospital seemed anomalous in a country that has 18% HIV prevalence compared to Kenya's 6%; but it was testament to the success of the work pioneered here: the people didn't have to come to hospital to be treated; 'the hospital' – in the form of family, neighbours and medical staff – went to them. This response had been so successful in reducing HIV/AIDS that Chikankata would become a template for other community HIV/AIDS response work around the world, a kind of international village to which doctors and professionals came to learn and take back the knowledge into their own communities.

We had come to see with our own eyes where the work had started and to talk to some of the people who had been here in those first days when a strange, arcane disease made its first appearance. For us, it was a necessary pilgrimage to the site of a significant battle in the war against the pandemic. And Captain Angela Hachitapika – who along with her husband was the senior officer stationed at the community – had been a key protagonist in the conflict.

I met her at her home, a hundred yards walk from the hospital where she had once worked as a nurse. We went and sat on chairs on the thick, spidery grass of her garden and I asked her to tell me the story of Chikankata. Angela was a measured, capable, intelligent woman – her talents had already taken her away from Chikankata to other territories and they would again (she and her husband were about to be promoted) – but I couldn't have had a more locally savvy and authoritative eyewitness. Born in Chikankata, she had lived here for most of her life and she had been there at the beginning of the HIV/AIDS epidemic. In 1986, Angela, then a young nurse at the Mission Hospital, was probably the first person to treat a case of AIDS at the hospital.

'I remember a man – a sick game ranger from the eastern province – who had come in with TB-like symptoms. The ranger had been through a number of hospitals but none of them had been able to help him. He had terrible sores on his mouth (they were in fact Karposi Sarcoma). People were saying "What is wrong with that man's mouth?" I decided to put the man on a trial of drugs to cure the TB but he had a severe reaction (something known as Stephen Johnson Syndrome) and although he recovered from the trial he died soon afterwards.'

After the ranger, staff at the hospital noticed that patients were presenting with tuberculosis of a different form: lymph nodes on both sides of the body rather than just one. They were resistant to treatment of the normal kind, extremely sick, and often dying within weeks. But the manner of their dying had the staff – including a young Australian doctor at the hospital, Dr Ian Campbell – thinking there was more to this man's death than TB. In those early days of the disease, the young Dr Campbell had been keeping a watchful eye on epidemiological developments, in particular a disease – then known as HTLV III – that seemed to be confined to the gay community in San Francisco, in the USA. The symptoms that were presenting in San Francisco were the same symptoms that they were beginning to see at Chikankata. Having heard that medical friends at the University Teaching Hospital were screening for HIV, Campbell decided to do some tests on the patients at Chikankata himself. The tests were random and fairly primitive, but in the few months after the appearance of the ranger, 27 patients tested positive.

'We didn't have a name for it at first,' Angela said.

Most days and in most places we went, it felt as if the pandemic had always been here; that it was the natural condition of a continent, a part of its life as old as any cultural practice. So it was a shock to hear someone recalling the days – only half her lifetime ago – when HIV/AIDS was something unknown, unnamed and yet to come. It was a jolting reminder that HIV/AIDS was a phenomenon barely out of its teens. The effects of its short, devastating life had been so far reaching and all pervasive that it was easy to forget this.

'There was a lot of fear around treating these patients; little was known about how the disease was transmitted and staff were afraid to handle them.'

The hospital had originally been established as a leprosy

hospital so there was capacity for isolating patients if necessary. But the successful switch to home-based care of leprosy had seen the isolation wards empty. Now those same wards were filling with a new, equally stigmatising and isolating disease and they were filling at a rate that the hospital could not accommodate. By 1987 it was clear that the medical community had to organise themselves. Initially the hospital tried to look at annexing these patients, but sheer numbers and the fact that people were sick for a long time saw them running out of space for the chronically ill.

The staff, knowing that family and community were central to everything that happened here, instinctively felt that a local community response was the only way forward. So they encouraged testees to bring family members with them for counselling, offering shared confidentiality. From there patients – even those who were dying – expressed a preference to go home.

'When we asked ourselves how we could support this, the idea for home-based care began.'

The hospital put up a team consisting of a social worker (who was really a counsellor) and a clinical officer (being between nurse and doctor they could prescribe medicine and, later, ARVs). They started to visit people in the community over a six-month period. The team used a yellow vehicle to do the visits. Most vehicles were white so when people saw the yellow vehicle they knew what it represented. People would ask: 'What are you doing?' and the response usually was 'We have been invited to visit a person in the home.' (Sending teams by invitation to the homes of the sick did more to destigmatise the issue of AIDS than any campaign could ever have done). The team visits told the community that someone was doing something about the disease that was beginning to affect everyone.

At about this time a London-based donor was offering funds to the hospital to effectively fill the leprosy wards with AIDS patients. But by now the medical staff at Chikankata were beginning to understand HIV and see their nascent programme of home-based care as the way forward. They didn't want to change the programme and were wary of throwing money and drugs at something so fragile. As new drugs came 'out-of-research gate', companies liked to test those drugs and would offer money for researching them. The team asked themselves what that would mean for the community and concluded that it was a short-term panacea that – unlike the home-based care – failed to consider the whole person's emotional and spiritual as well as physical needs. They said no to the idea of institutionalising people with AIDS and pressed on with their plan.

Another significant moment in the formation of the work happened at the end of 1987 when Doctor Campbell and his staff were invited to a community near the Zambezi River in a dry, drought affected area of the Gwembe valley. The son of a headman had killed himself by burning his hut down after discovering that he was HIV positive. The headman knew his son had been visited by the hospital team and he asked the team to come and talk to his community. He wanted to know more about this disease but he wanted more than information.

'Don't just treat us; educate us,' he said. 'Help us think.'

This visit and the conversation it instigated was the beginning of a counselling process that grew into the community conversations that we had seen at work in Kenya and Uganda. By the end of 1987 a community driven care and prevention response, supported by care and conversation at the hospital, had become the accepted method of responding to HIV/AIDS in Chikankata.

What was remarkable about this approach was that it lead to change in cultural practices that had gone on for years; practices that the pandemic exposed and amplified. The model built on the extended family system and encouraged the community to take responsibility for sick relatives themselves. Through the conversations, the people began to question certain practices, in particular the sexual cleansing of widows or ritual cleansing. In ritual cleansing, after a death of a husband or wife, the surviving spouse was supposed to undergo a custom with a family member of the deceased, and often this took the form of one episode of sexual intercourse sometime during the prolonged funeral. It was seen as a way of exorcising the spirit of death from the widowed person. In the new paradigm of HIV/AIDS this was a disaster. It usually meant a woman – whose husband had died of HIV/AIDS and who was most likely infected herself – having intercourse with someone who was already married to at least one wife. But the community counselling process* saw people challenging the practice. Soon, even the chiefs (many of them with more than one wife) came out in favour of abolishing it. Simple though it sounds, this was the first significant example of family and neighbourhood driven care and concern that led to risk reduction through behavioural change. And in early 1990 all the headmen of the area, numbering over one hundred, met to agree on a local by-law to ban ritual cleansing by sexual intercourse. Later in the year this decision was transferred to a meeting of chiefs in Lusaka and the by-law was introduced for the whole country.

Change. So easy to say; so hard to bring about. In all the systems of measuring the relative success of the fight against AIDS, change was the hardest thing to measure. For Angela change was really the difference between treating the problem and defeating it. And the exciting thing was that seemingly small advances in practice were seismic in cultural terms; and they were highly infectious, leading to changes in other, perhaps more subtle and ubiquitous, practices.

'For instance,' Angela explained: 'traditionally a wife was not

---

* In a study conducted through the hospital, it was found that without family counselling in the home setting, 50% of families carried on with the custom that obviously carried risk of transmission of HIV; yet with family counselling 90% of families did not carry out the custom in that way; instead they chose a more traditional form of custom, such as jumping over a cow or a line at the funeral.

allowed to touch a husband if he was sick – it had to be done by his own blood relative and vice versa, a man could not take care of his sick wife. "Go and get your mother," he would say. AIDS and the Care Prevention Teams had flipped that practice on its head. Now wives are able to touch their sick husbands. Now you actually see men sit on the bedside, as well as the mother, sometimes instead of the mother.'

'What about the traditionalists?' I asked Angela. 'Do they think these changes are bad?'

'They should know already, from their traditions, that "Trouble of your friend today will be trouble on you tomorrow."'

The care extended through the response had the two-way effect of sifting what was healthy and what was malignant in the existing culture.

'And have things really changed?'

'Of course. There is no more sexual cleansing and wife inheritance is decreasing. One man one wife is more common. Whole families now come for VCT (voluntary counselling and testing). People who are not biologically connected look after one another. And, men are fully involved in the caring business! That never used to happen. Even the men. I saw a man with a baby on his back today. There! An African man carrying a baby! That is real change.'

So is it fair to say that Chikankata's story shows that an organic, indigenous response can work better than many externally prescribed responses and that communities are better than service organizations at solving their issues?'

Angela had no doubts about this: 'Let's go back to the community. That is how we have managed here. I don't need an NGO to pay me for my needs. Here in Zambia – and in Africa – health and life is communal not individual. The answer to our problems lies in understanding this truth.'

The Smoke That Thunders

'What shall I do with this sad situation?'
– lyric from '*Todii*', a song, by Zimbabwe musician
Oliver Mtukudzi, about someone living with
HIV/AIDS

At the Victoria Falls border crossing bridge you can walk half way across and stand with one foot in Zambia and one foot in Zimbabwe. There is a sign there that says: 'You are now entering Zimbabwe' and there was a day – maybe ten years ago – when it was possible to read the sign without interpreting threat in the statement. Back then the sign would have filled the traveller with a sense of excitement that they were crossing from relatively poor Zambia to rich Zimbabwe, a country so productive and bountiful it was called 'The Breadbasket of Africa'. Now, according to reports, Zimbabwe had become The Breadbasketcase of Africa: a sad, maddening place with a plummeting life expectancy and rocketing inflation,* ruled by a bitter and malignant dictator whose ruination of the economy had left the country's flour mills barely able to provide bread for its own people, let alone the rest of the continent.

At the bridge, clusters of money exchangers skulked with doorstep wads of Zim Dollars looking to change for Zambian Kwatcha. The men were from Zimbabwe but had 'escaped' to

---

* At the time of going to press, Zimbabwe's inflation was at 1700%.

Zambia to seek a better life; or perhaps a longer life than the 39 years the average Zimbabwean is now expected to live. We were heading the other way and were going to need some Zim money for our bus journey (our US dollars were not viable there – as all foreign currency was banned). Exchanging money with these men was chancy; not because they were mendacious, but because it was impossible to work out a competitive rate. Just across that bridge, beyond the sign, there was a nation in the grip of the world's highest inflation. At the time of passage, war-torn Iraq's inflation – the world's second highest – stood at 80%; Zimbabwe's stood at 1400%.

Captain Kennedy, from the Salvation Army in Lusaka, had escorted us here and he took our Kwatcha (about fifty pounds worth) and used his imposing physique and good humour to negotiate a fair rate with the men. He came back with fresh, pink wads of 50,000 Zim dollar notes that looked like the booty from a major bank robbery.

'Here,' he said handing me two tied stacks. 'That's about thirty million. That will buy you a soda over there on the other side.'

The mist from the spray from the falls shrouded the view across the border towards Zimbabwe. The Victoria Falls had been dutifully named after an English queen by the explorer who 'discovered' them, but this dull moniker was no match for the local name – *Mosi Oa Tunya* – that roughly translates as 'The Smoke That Thunders'. Standing on that bridge, we could see the smoke spray and feel it on our skin and hear the thunder of the bubbling gorge below. The sudden crash of the Zambezi into the gorge produced a sight so wonderful that for a moment you could forget about the trouble across the bridge.

Later, at a border crossing, all the passengers from our bus joined a long queue made up of people who had already disembarked from the buses up ahead. About two hundred people stretched back from the customs hut and remained shade-less until it reached the veranda of the hut – a journey the man next to me judged to be about an hour. Nicola and the children went to find cover from the midday sun and I did the first shift in the queue, talking to the tall, smartly dressed Zimbabwean who had just completed a three-year-degree at Durham University in England.

'So what is over that bridge?' I asked him.

'A beautiful country in big trouble.'

'Are things as bad as they say?'

'The reports do not lie,' he said.

The reports he meant were the ones he'd read and watched in England; the same reports I was relying on for my own information and from which I had built up a picture of a country in the very process of collapsing. In the hour it took to get from the exposed road and the covered hut, my tall Shona friend and I covered a lot of ground. He explained that Zimbabwe was essentially made up of two tribal groups, the Shona and the Ndebele. The Shona were seen as peaceful; the Ndebele more forceful. The Shona were the numerically dominant tribe and mainly in the north, the Ndebele were in the south. Robert Mugabe was Shona. When I asked the man how much longer people would put up with the situation, he told me that Zimbabweans were gentle people and that made them long suffering. They would rather wait till things got better than change things by force.

'If this was Nigeria,' he said, 'there would have been blood by now.'

We were almost in the hut when he asked me why we were entering Zimbabwe at a time such as this. I felt I could trust him, but I was wary of mentioning my own reporting credentials, particularly the three-letter acronym so reviled by the Zimbabwe's leadership. I had been advised, by the BBC World Service, not to do any recording with my mini-disc and had buried it amongst our underwear with the big truncheon microphone in the hidden compartment of my rucksack. If I was found to be doing anything for the BBC in Zimbabwe it could get me thrown out of the country or land me in jail. The advice I got from the Salvation Army regional team was to keep my eyes and ears on the AIDS response work and not delve into the politics.

'I'm a writer,' I said. 'I'm here to look at the AIDS work the Salvation Army are doing.' I asked him if he had any relatives with AIDS, knowing there would be a one in five chance of this in a country with 26% prevalence.

'Everyone here has relatives with AIDS.'

On the wall, just inside the entrance to the customs hut, there was a poster admonishing us – the people? the government? – to stamp out corruption. Once in the hut, under the gaze of the customs guards, we ceased our chat about the state of the nation and I found myself policing my thoughts, just in case the guards saw them hanging in the air like think bubbles.

What I was thinking was: why are we paying more than everyone else to enter this country? And: shall I risk asking the question for fear that any subversion might delay our passage? Every non-national entering Zimbabwe that day paid a visa fee of 35 US dollars (and it needed to be paid in US dollars). We – being British citizens – paid 55 US dollars. I knew exactly why we were paying twenty dollars more than the rest of mankind, but I wanted to make sure that it was the piece of petty revenge I suspected and not just some bureaucratic oversight.

'Why are we were paying more than other human beings coming to Zimbabwe?' I asked the customs official through the half glass partition.

The official laughed at me.

'You are British. The government do not like you. So you must pay extra.'

He stamped our four passports and handed them back with a crocodile smile: 'Welcome to Zimbabwe.'

We arrived at the Salvation Army compound in Harare in darkness. The state grid was load sharing electric power and it was the western part of the city's turn to go without light for two hours. Our driver – a captain from the Harare Corps – used the headlights of the vehicle to illuminate the house that was to be our base and launch pad for our stay in Zimbabwe. Inside, we strapped the 'pit latrine' torches to our heads, lit the candles and looked around. Even with the lights switched off, it was easy to see that this country had reached a level of economic development and possessed an infrastructure way above that of a Kenya or a Uganda. The house was spacious, well made and well appointed; it had a fridge, bath and shower and (most of the day) power. It was hard to countenance that, out there, beyond the gates, there was a people enduring the lowest life expectancy in the world.

Later, when the lights came on, and we had eaten our three million dollar pizzas kindly delivered by Colonel Bob Ward, we sat in front of the television and watched the news on Zimbabwe's only terrestrial channel – the state-owned ZTV. It was an uninformative but very telling experience. We joined at the international news segue and a feature on the opening of the Three Gorges Dam in China. The tone was glowing and awestruck. This item was followed by a piece about a medical breakthrough in China. And then a piece about China's trade relations with African nations. Between the lines of these dull, irrelevant features you could detect the real story: the look east policy of a government cutting free from 'colonial masters' and looking for solace in a relationship with one of the few countries in the world who didn't treat it as a pariah.

There was then a news item in which the vice president Joyce Majura was seen touring farms in Zimbabwe. The vice president – who regularly attended a Salvation Army church in Harare and who I had ambitiously sought an interview with because of this – was shown giving a speech in which she was saying that the agricultural problem needed to be solved fast. Since the 'land grab' agriculture had gone into rapid decline; even if the land grab was fair, as was possible to argue, the management of the land since had been a shambles. To see a Zimbabwean politician saying as much was a relief; what wasn't said was that it was the government who created the problem in the first place by giving the land as favours to a few people with no expertise in farming. It was hard to work out: was Majura going as far as she could to criticise Mugabe without naming him? Or was she doing what Mugabe did and blaming everyone else but the government for the economic decline of Zimbabwe?

After the news, the viewing swung from the bland to the shrill as we watched a thrillingly inappropriate quiz show called 'Money or the Box'. The show's jovial host must have been beaming from a parallel universe of unconcern to have pulled his presentation off with such cheery aplomb. This was a show where – because of inflation – there were 'literally billions of dollars to be won!' As well as cash prizes rendered silly by the current economic state of that nation, there were mystery prizes in the box: holidays, household furniture, cars. The contestants were whittled down until one man was left to choose his prize. His choice was between a cash prize of several million Zim dollars or what was in the box – potentially a holiday for two in South Africa or a car. The lucky man chose the box. When you're living in a country where people risk swimming across the crocodile infested Limpopo River to escape to South Africa, who's going to turn down a potential free flight out?

Whenever we arrived in a new country (a territory in Salvation Army parlance) we would follow a pattern of procedure that usually started with 'orientation' – a settling in, followed by a presentation of an itinerary of our visit and a budget of costs. There would then be a courtesy meeting with the Territorial Commander, if he or she was available. In the case of Zimbabwe, our itinerary had been planned a number of weeks before our arrival – at a time when inflation was a mere 1000%. The proposal we were shown in that first meeting involved an ambitious two-week immersion in three communities at almost diametrically opposite ends of what is a country twice the size of France. It would mean over 2500 miles driving in two weeks and the estimated cost for the visit was – at the newly adjusted rate of exchange – close to 2800 US dollars.

We had so far stuck with the Salvation Army's judgement on what needed to be seen and how far we needed to go to see it; but this was too much. Even without the costs (which was nearly all for gasoline) this schedule was a big ask for the family and for the first time in the whole trip we baulked.

'We can't do this amount of travelling. Can we compress it – do two of the three?'

The team were slightly thrown by this but Stanford – the senior officer in the meeting – said they could cut out the thousand mile round trip to Thselanyemba in the southern reaches of the country. Instead he suggested we could see some of the work nearer to Harare and make a visit to Howard Hospital, about fifty miles north of the city.

'That sounds good,' I said. 'And maybe we could see where the refugees are after the bulldozing of the slum areas last year?'

This suggestion was met with nervous laughter.

'There is nothing to see. Those people are not there any more.'

On our way to visit Howard Hospital, an hour out of the city, Nicola and I decided to ask our escort – two female Zimbabwean officers – about 'Operation Murambatsvina' (Operation Clean Up Filth). We wanted to know (because we had heard about it and seen footage in our own country) about the demolition of the 'slum' areas of Harare carried out by the government the year before and what the Salvation Army had done about the resulting homelessness of the de-housed people.

The answer we got wasn't what you'd expect to hear from someone in the Salvation Army. 'Those people were crooks. Thieves. They were selling things illegally. Causing trouble.'

'But we saw on the news – on the BBC – pictures of bulldozed housing and ordinary people living in shells, saying they had nowhere to go. They did not look like crooks. Many of the people in those slums were poor families, including many people with HIV.'

'You should not believe those reports. They have their own agenda.'

The second officer nodded emphatically in agreement and said: 'Yes. You don't know in your country what is really happening.'

'But we have a free press. You don't have a free press here.'

'That is not true. We have a free press.'

This was an alarming exchange. We were sitting in the back of the car and we looked at each other wondering how to proceed.

Nicola wasn't having it.

'I thought the Salvation Army ministered to people without prejudice. Shouldn't you have helped those people? Shouldn't you have made a protest? '

'Most people were happy at what happened because those people were making trouble for everyone else. Now they have all gone back to their farms in the countryside. Things are much better.'

'You mean back to their farms which have been ruined by this government's policy of taking over land?'*

Again smiles and laughter at our apparent lack of correct information on this subject.

'That is not the government's fault.'

'But those people left their farms because they came looking for work because there was no longer work on the farms because they'd been badly managed.'

---

* The land grab by colonialists in the 1930s is at the root of the land grab by Mugabe.

'I think you cannot believe all these things. Yes there are some problems with the farming.'

'Some problems! It has been a disaster.'

'Things are not so bad as you think. The government are trying to change it. They are trying to get those farms working.'

'But they're not working. And people are going hungry. People don't have food. Or money for food.'

'It is not as bad as this. There are many troublemakers just interested in stirring things up. They say these things just to get into power.'

'So it's not true? That people are suffering because of this government?'

'The government cannot be blamed for everything.'

We stopped asking questions after this. George Orwell once wrote that when you live under a dictatorship, you train yourself not to see things in order to survive. Maybe this was such a case.

It was a relief to get to Howard Hospital. To get back to AIDS. Ah yes, the purpose of our visit. I had almost forgotten. Don't get involved in the politics. Keep your eyes and ears on the AIDS work and maybe you'll see the link between the situation in the country and the daily struggles on the ground. If you want to find out how a country is really doing talk to a doctor.

Howard was led by a talented, unusual, Canadian doctor who had lived here for years and married a Zimbabwean.

'So, doctor. How much of your work here is AIDS related?'

'If there was no AIDS, I'd be practically unemployed.' HIV/AIDS related illness and opportunistic infections took up about 60–70% of his work.

I wanted to know how politics affected the HIV/AIDS situation on the ground.

'Traditionally the work here has been donor supported. One aspect of the problems in the country is the decline of donor support.'

'And has this exacerbated the problems?'

'Well actually, on the ground we've seen that small organisations can do a lot with little.'

'So you have managed?'

'Our mission response has improved because it has had to. When you're in a tight corner you have to think quick about how to respond. Ten years ago we were hospital-centric. Now we have more community volunteers using whatever resources they can muster to look after patients with HIV. We provide some things – training, logistics, soap – but the volunteers provide the psycho-support and do the real work. It proves what we already suspected: that the top down approach to AIDS simply is not sustainable.'

If I was planning to show some kind of link between bad politics and worsening HIV then I wasn't going to find it here. And in truth, I was glad. Glad that what we had seen at work in other parts of Africa – 'the bottom up approach' – was robust enough to withstand all manner of catastrophe. Once again, it was the little guys and not the big chiefs who were keeping it all going.

On the way out we had a quick look at the dispensary. This was where the ARVs were kept and it was the first time we had actually seen ARVs like this anywhere. The nurse showed us how many packets were needed for one person's daily consumption. It was an enormous stack, although she said the drug companies had already managed to get it down by 50% in the last two years.

'You have enough drugs?'

'There is no shortage of drugs here; the problem is having enough food to absorb the drugs. Right now, that's a problem.'

In the next few days – while we waited for permission to go on our trip north – tricky conversations suddenly became non-conversations. People were polite but the indigenous members of the Salvation Army seemed reluctant to discuss anything to do with the situation in their country. At first I put this down to what the man at the border had said: that Zimbabweans were non-confrontational, waiting for trouble to pass on. But it was to prove more insidious than that. It felt more and more that people were afraid to talk about it or, worse, they had been ordered not to. Or maybe they didn't really have any idea. Was it possible that the Salvation Army here was living in a protective bubble? They had always been in the front line of things – but here in Harare the corps was more established and more 'establishment'. Indeed, they were established enough for some senior members of government to be counted as church members. Maybe this was part of the problem.

To get around the silence I eschewed the Corps' minibus ride into the HQ of the Salvation Army and took taxis. I wanted to connect with people, outside the gates. I walked to the nearest supermarket, along William Booth Road, past people selling vegetables and fruit from makeshift 'stores' and people waiting for minibus rides into the centre of town. It looked, at first, like the normal everyday activity of a major African city. I bought an apple from a woman selling fruit. She was stirring a pot on a stove. The pot contained a porridge-like mealy maize and two other women sat with her topping and tailing green beans and throwing them into the pot.

'How are things?' I asked.

'Things are very difficult.' The woman said. 'We have no money for rent,' the woman said. 'We are living here now.'

'Where?'

'Here.' 'Here' was a fruit stall with a bivouac. Were these women the 'filth' the government meant when they launched their clean-up operation?

I went on to the supermarket to buy a newspaper. The supermarket had installed special counting machines to cope with the super escalation of inflation and the amount of notes required to purchase simple items. The people queued with carrier bags full of money. The cruel trick of this inflation was that it created the illusion that you had a lot of money. One day you had millions, the next day nothing.

I purchased a newspaper – *The Herald* – and then went to the taxi rank. Operating on the universal law that taxi drivers had opinions and shared them, I decided that I would take as many taxi rides as possible and put together a tape of some kind based on interviews with taxi drivers, in the hope that at least someone in this country might tell me what life was really like. My first driver was an apologist for his government.

'How do you feel about the situation in your country?' I asked him.

'I'm not a political commentator,' he said.

'But do you feel free to criticise the government,' I ask him.

'There is some criticism.'

'Where?'

'In the news. They are allowed to report things.'

'Where?'

He couldn't answer me.

I read him the story from the day's state-owned *Herald*. 'Here. There's a story about Robert Mugabe. He has sworn in new commissioners as part of his plan to change the parliamentary election to coincide with presidential elections so he'll rule until 2010. And there is not any criticism of this move. Not even anyone asking the question – is this okay?'

He went on to say, in a semi-defence of what was happening, that the government here was only doing what other African post-colonial governments were doing and trying to adopt their own system of government not influenced by the West. Like Uganda.

'Like a big boss – big chief – system,' I asked. 'Where one man rules forever?'

'The trouble is they want power for a long time. That is not good,' he admitted.

Then his phone went and he took the call.

The next taxi driver was melancholy.

'Life. How are you finding it?' I asked.

'Things are difficult. You get salary, make one shopping trip, buy soap, toothpaste. No money left. 90% of people are suffering.'

'Everyone except the people in the government?'

(We were driving close to the opulent Presidential palace, past the armed guards and sealed-off roads. Past the cricket ground and the sports club and golf course).

He nodded. 'You know what the joke they are saying. The problem with Zimbabwe? It's the IMF.'

'The IMF? Why?'

'Is Mugabe's Fault.'

'What are the people going to do about it?'

'People are just tired. Hoping it will just go away, as long as you get your meal.'

'Is something going to happen?'

'I think nothing will happen. Stalemate. The people are hopeless, powerless.'

'Do you think if the government changes things will get better?'

'Maybe but the issue is management of economy. So we can do more than just survive.'

The third taxi driver was despairing.

'We used to eat but now we don't have the money.'

'I'm sorry.'

'It's really tough. I've been working overnight, trying to make my children survive. I have two in school.'

'You've been living in Zim all your life. Was it this bad during the war?'

'It was much better during wartime. We have peace now but bad economics.'

'Do you feel free?'

'You don't feel free when you don't have anything to eat.'

It was time to meet the chief of the Salvation Army in Zimbabwe. Our meeting with the Territorial Commander had been delayed because he had been where, I later learned, he had had to answer some difficult questions about the situation in his country, back at the International Headquarters in London. He greeted me and ushered me to sit.

'So,' he asked, in an avuncular way, 'how are you finding things here in Zimbabwe?'

Oddly, his tone was that of a man confident that his guest had landed in a paradise of tranquillity and was going to be full of nothing but praise. Despite this, I didn't think there was any harm in me being honest with my answer, even if it meant sounding disappointed and even ungrateful to my totemic host. This man was on my side, after all. He was a Christian, he was engaged in helping those in need, he knew what was going on out there.

'To be honest I have found things quite difficult. It is hard to talk to people here about the situation. So, I have been talking to taxi drivers. And shop keepers. For this BBC tape.'

'Those people will say things.'

'Yes. They all said pretty much the same thing. Things are very bad. It can't go on much longer. When will it end?'

The switch from a welcoming greeting to the defensive was instant.

'You must listen to me. I am not happy that you are doing this recordings for the BBC. Do you know what will happen if the government knew that we had someone from the BBC here?'

'I am not from the BBC; I am a freelance writer, on my own, trying to tell the story of what I see. The BBC is just one thing I am doing work for. But mainly I am writing a book about the AIDS work the Salvation Army are doing around the world.'

'I was told you were here to see the good work we are doing with HIV/AIDS.'

'Yes… I want to see the AIDS work but I have to ask the

question – how this work is affected by the situation in your country. They are not separate.'

'So why did you ask to interview Joyce Majura?'

'It seemed like a question worth asking. It raised some important issues: how a woman – anyone actually – could hold in tension two such seemingly antagonistic positions. How a church and its members adjusted to tyranny.'

'This is not possible. You need to understand I need to protect the church here. '

'But what if the government act against the principles of the church?'

He was not happy with me.

'Let me tell you how it is. You do not understand how it is. We have to be very careful. When you go to the AIDS community work in Hurungwe, you must not use the recorder, or take any photographs there. You will meet the chief; he is also a government agent. And they are having local elections up there. It is dangerous for you to stay there.'

'Is it safe for me to take the family?'

'It is okay but you must not stay there.'

'But it's six hundred miles. How can I see the work if we have an hour. And I don't want my children sitting in a car all day.'

'You cannot stay there,' he repeated. 'You might stay at the border. I will talk to them.'

Silence. I didn't want to be there. I had upset him and he me. I could see his point of view; that this was a difficult situation for him. And he was grappling with a complex history.

'This was a great country. We were the breadbasket of the whole continent. And we will be a great nation again. Too many come to look for trouble stories. And the BBC and the Western press they say these things. The BBC put out their own propaganda, making it sound much worse and that does not help anything.'

It was an echo of the conversation in the car going to Howard Hospital; but this was a territorial commander telling me that a news organisation I worked for was putting out lies. Pride in country is fine, to a point, but this was something else. I had no puff left for argument. His remarks had the effect of a blow out. I lost my bearings for a second and couldn't keep my self on the road. Thankfully, he stood up and reverted to the tone of greeting he'd adopted at the beginning.

'Well, it has been good meeting you. I hope you have a good journey to the Hurungwe community.'

We shook hands and I left.

I walked straight out of the headquarters and down to a café in a smart, clientless, boutique shopping mall, about a hundred yards from the headquarters. I bought a latte for 300,000 dollars and sat there going over the encounter in my mind, bit by bit, checking that I had heard it right, got it right, got him right.

What I had heard, or thought I'd heard, was a man in a position of eminence in an international organisation telling me that my understanding was limited because I came from a country whose press (a press I did occasionally work for) was not interested in reporting truth when he himself lived in a country which patently did not have a free press. What I thought I'd heard was a man who should be on the pulse of events telling me his country was going to be a great country again, one of the greatest in Africa, when in fact it had slipped in twenty years from a position of pre-eminence to bottom place in almost every league table of wellbeing you could muster.

I told myself to put myself in his shoes. Maybe there were things he could not tell me and that his position was more compromised than I realised and than he was able to say. Maybe he was a proud Zimbabwean and this country was still, relatively speaking, emerging from its colonial past, a past that was a kind of disgrace in itself. Maybe it might just be possible for someone living in a country without a free press – even a person of relative seniority – to be ignorant of what was going on. I tried to remember what I had seen almost everywhere we'd been: the Salvation Army were superbly disciplined about not judging events and people.

But I was too upset to be gracious. How could he not know? A man in such a position should know better. I had seen, just the day before on the internet, a BBC report, interviewing people made homeless in Operation Clean Up: were these people making it up? And why the little speech about Zimbabwe being a great country again? What did greatness mean in his eyes, a man who lived by a different standard and had a different measuring system for success?

I started to wonder if I had – we had, the West had – actually got it all wrong; that the reports of food shortages and inflation were exaggerated by outside agencies in order to unsettle the government. That the things the taxi drivers and fruit stall sellers were saying were not to be trusted. That the levels of HIV/AIDS – among the highest in the world – were made up, too.

I checked myself. This is what a lack of freedom does to the mind. It stops it from thinking clearly. Oppression wants to confuse you. It wants you to not be sure of anything. By creating uncertainty and then offering itself as the only certainty. Fear is subtle. It chips away at clear thinking until it distorts reality, making it hard to assess the situation as it really is. Were we actually in danger? Maybe. Two other people told me that if government agents knew that I had any connection to the BBC and was doing work here, I would be taken in for questioning. Someone else said that the phones in the compound were bugged. Zimbabwe is in such a poor state it hardly seemed likely they'd have a special police force capable of tracking me down. Policemen were surely too busy worrying about what everyone else was worrying about: where the next meal was coming from. But tyranny gets a free ride from the fear it induces; it doesn't have to do all the policing because it gets people to police themselves and that is what it felt like in Zimbabwe; simply trying to survive had enervated the people; damping down any righteous inclination to do anything about it; fear did the rest.

Across the mini piazza, a music shop was playing a beautiful, melancholy tune. I went into the shop and asked the man what it was. He showed me the CD case. It was by Oliver Mtukudzi and the song was called 'Todii'.

'He is a great Zimbabwean songwriter,' the man said.

The words to the song repeated over and over: 'Todii…what shall we do…(about this sad situation).' The man said the song was all about HIV/AIDS and the sleeve notes confirmed this. The song was written from the point of view of someone living with HIV. I asked to listen to some more tracks, including one called Magumo: 'How will it all end?' The song asked the question over and over: 'What will be the end of all this?' According to the sleeve notes, the song was about 'people who have power and money and do not respect those who are physically and socially weak.'

AIDS and political oppression are first cousins, with similar characteristics: they both use fear to perpetuate themselves, they silence the sufferer and hit the people least able to cope harder than anyone else.

I bought the CD, using up the last of my pink 50,000 notes I'd exchanged on the black market and caught a taxi back to the compound, singing to myself the question:

'What shall we do?'

What we did was get up at five the next morning to make the long trek north to the border where a communal HIV/AIDS response had just been established in a community that was non-Christian and run on the old tribal lines. Our visit meant meeting the chief who was – as the TC had suggested – more than likely a government agent. This was not as sinister as it sounded; most chiefs were approached by the government to get their people to vote in a particular way in exchange for concessions. But it added to the sense of danger. As we had seen on ZTV, there had already been some trouble in the south, where votes against Zanu PF had been seen as 'rigged' and opposition leaders had been put under house arrest for 'attempting to subvert the peace'.

Our driver seemed unhappy. All evening there had been a flurry of calls: the trip was on; the trip was off. We were allowed to stay overnight; we were not allowed to stay. At the last hour, Marguerite Ward, Bob's wife who ran the HIV programme, had insisted we make the trip and got an officer to take us there. What was not clear was whether we'd be staying overnight or not. The officer did not seem to know himself. He remained quite silent for the entire six hundred mile journey. He was – I had been told – a friendly and jovial man, but I think by now the Brook family were giving off a bad stench (both our previous accompaniments had suddenly dropped out of the programme).

Our journey broke half way at the house of a Major and the regional team organiser who had made the connection with the chief and the community in Hurungwe. The Major – recently widowed – had prepared a breakfast for us himself. He and his assistant were welcoming and their friendliness only served to exaggerate the cold-shouldering we'd been getting in Harare. We ate our breakfast of eggs and bread and jam and fruit. The captain then fielded a call on his mobile. He looked perturbed. He handed the phone to the Major. It was from headquarters. We were not to stay in the community, but to return that same day. The TC had intervened. Either the TC knew something he couldn't share, or he was just not trusting me to obey his prohibition. Was he protecting us or just not trusting us? No reason was given.

We drove on to the community, another 150 miles into the bush. It was beautiful landscape but our mood was tainted by the knowledge that we'd have to drive back that same day and that our stay was becoming untenable. Through that prism, the scenery was hard to appreciate.

We eventually reached a collection of pointed straw and mud houses on a mud-packed sight, with a chieftain's meeting *kraal* at its heart. This elegant construction was raised up high on the stilts of thick trunks of wood, away from the termites and ants. Three men were in its shade, including the chief who wore a leather cow hat and sat in a big armchair, also leather. If I'd been allowed to I would have taken a picture.

Our party joined him, the chief's son pulling up little stools for us to sit on. The Major translated his words of greeting. The chief was intrigued to see that I had come with my children. This impressed him. The chief said he had many children by three wives (each of the huts around the *kraal* contained a wife). The chief asked, through his son, why I had come here. He did not look directly at me when he spoke, although I knew he was watching me. I confirmed what I knew he had been told: that I was here to see the good work the community were doing in responding to HIV/AIDS.

Maybe I was still smarting from the news that another kind of chief had ordered our return home that day but I began to feel irritated at this tribal protocol; and all these big chiefs running the show; annoyed with *this* chief who wouldn't quite look at me, and who was in cahoots with a government, and who had three wives. I felt that my well of goodwill had run dry in these last few days. Why do we have to jump through these hoops? Why do old men with potbellies and shifty eyes, who practice polygamy and prop up other bad chiefs get to call the shots?

But we moved on and the chief, to his credit, came along too. It was the first time he had been to such a meeting. He said he wanted to sit in on the community conversation because AIDS was a big problem and everyone needed to be at the meeting, him included. One of his wives came with him to another hot hut with a corrugated tin roof where we were greeted by the gathered community. We spoke about the work we'd seen (the Major translated) and we talked about HIV/AIDS and soon we began to engage again with people and actually have a conversation. Despite the chief's presence, people spoke very freely and the chief himself prompted a greater degree of questioning. In the two hours that we were there we almost forgot where we were. To hear these people talking about sex, about faithfulness, about stigma – just to have a full conversation – was a tonic after the muzzled experience of Harare.

We had been told how good the community response was in Zimbabwe by April Foster and by the regional response youth leader, Meble Birengo, in Nairobi. Meble was a wise and highly gifted twenty-five-year-old who had seen the work close up in most countries. Her opinion counted so we had been saddened and frustrated at not being able to see what she meant. The strength of the response here was lost – for us – in the politics of it all. However, these few hours in Hurungwe redeemed something for us. Towards the end of the meeting, one bright and lively young man stood up to speak. He was full of ideas about how to tackle AIDS. He had started a football team for the orphans and they trained together every week. They needed football kit – some of them had no shirts – but this team had made everyone notice the size of the problem. A whole team of orphans! He said that the biggest problem for their community had been not talking about HIV/AIDS. People pretended that it would somehow go away if they didn't talk about it. But the opposite is true, he said. 'Sooner or later you have to face the thing you don't want to talk about.'

On the way back to Harare we decided that we should leave Zimbabwe as soon as possible. Our visit was causing problems and the BBC connection was a dangerous one. People talk – yes, even people who go to church – and there were people in the church here who were one degree of separation away from government. An incident the next day, as I set off for headquarters to say we were leaving, confirmed that it was time. As I passed through the compound checkpoint, the young guard at the gate – a guard I not seen before – said hello. I said hello back and then he said: 'You're the guy from the BBC.'

I said, no. I was with the Salvation Army.

'Oh.' He said and he smiled at me. 'I heard you were.'

'Heard from whom?'

He shrugged. It could have been an innocent enough exchange. Someone had said something to someone else and now that someone had said something to a guard.

But it was signal enough. It was time to go.

Our experience in Zimbabwe and our ability to see the AIDS response work there had been severely compromised by the political situation but also by our own choice not to see all of the good work that there was there to see. In hindsight, this was our loss. It was also made more difficult by my connections to the BBC; a fact that put particular strain on the leadership of the Salvation Army in Harare. They had the delicate job of protecting themselves and us; something we were probably not as fully appreciative of as we should have been at the time. The criticism in my account comes as much from a frustration at what we could not see, as from what we could.

In Rudyard Kipling's *The Elephant's Child,* the young elephant, who suffers from a surfeit of 'satiable curiosity', is sent by his increasingly irritable relatives down to the great grey greasy banks of the Limpopo River (now a geographical borderline between South Africa and Zimbabwe) to get the answers to his questions. And it is there that the elephant gets an answer to his awkward question from the crocodile that latches on to his nose. In his attempt to escape from the crocodile the elephant gets his trunk. After a few days in Zimbabwe, I had begun to feel like that Elephant Child: whenever I asked a question it was either met with a rueful deflecting smile or a sighing grumpiness; the people I was asking either didn't know the answers or didn't want to think about it. I had travelled with the mantra of 'Ask the naïve questions and you'll get somewhere close to the truth' in mind but Zimbabwe was to prove a challenging place to do this. The people here had stopped asking the questions because they were too busy trying to survive or because they were afraid. What we didn't expect was the Salvation Army to play the part of the grumpy and protective relative and send us – a few weeks later – across the Limpopo River with so many questions unanswered.

Who's the Daddy Now?

We drove across the Limpopo River and into South Africa, through Kruger and on to the Johannesburg freeway. The roads and the cars and the buildings and the food and the coffee told us we'd entered a country at an entirely different level of economic development to anything else we'd encountered in Africa. Entering South Africa felt like leaving Africa.

In Johannesburg we passed tall, shining office towers and the artificial hills of the city's gold mines, along the N-3 freeway towards Soweto. Somewhere ahead there was a city of two million people. Eventually we came to an exit sign (not so long ago Soweto wasn't even on the map) and moments later Soweto appeared: a vast, undifferentiated sprawl of little homes sitting in a shallow valley. It was hard to associate this sleepy, bland mass with such a bright, violent past. That incendiary history was now a market for tourists who came here to see the townships, art galleries and museums. By the standards of other African city sub-cities, Soweto was salubrious. The new burgeoning, black middle-classes were moving in rather than out.

We stayed with Nomsa – a friend of our accompanying Captain – and her house on the corner of Crossroads, right in the heart of the township, stood out like a statement. Nomsa was a strong, proud woman who had built up a successful grocery business. She now had a chain of three stores and plans for more. She had achieved her success single-handedly and her house – with its marble floors, televisions in every room, electric garage, heavy ornate furnishings, plunge bath – was an expression of her independence and self-made pride. 'Look, I did this, me a single woman in Soweto,' it declared. Another African woman getting by without the support of a husband.

We were joined for dinner by Ricardo Walters, the Salvation Army's regional team co-ordinator. Ricardo was – like April Foster and Dr Ian Campbell and Mark Mutungwa and others involved in the regional response team – part of the Salvation Army, but distinct from it. He wore pretty slick clothes and he had no rank – as far as I knew. Ricardo, like many of the people involved in the AIDS work was part of the Army but separate. AIDS had forced the regular Salvation Army to find other ways, other people, to reach those it traditionally thought it needed to reach. But if Ricardo didn't dress like a Salvationist he still had red, yellow and blue blood coursing through his veins.* His parents (as with April's and Mark's and almost everyone we met working in the field) were both members of the Salvation Army. It said something that so many children of Salvationists grew up to be active Salvationists themselves. I looked hard, but never once met a lapsed Salvationist on the entire journey. When I put this observation to April she said it was because 'most Salvation Army kids grew up seeing their parents doing the stuff they said they believed in, as opposed to just talking about it, and it made sense to do the same.'

At dinner, we talked about the recent history of Soweto and the days when it had the less musical name of South West Township. We talked about riots and curfews, of the bad days and the even worse days and then of Mandela and the end of apartheid. Mandela led us to AIDS via the death of his son and how it took this event to get the people at the top taking AIDS seriously. South Africa proved that you don't have to be oppressed to be in denial; the government – maybe distracted by other things

---

* The colours of the Salvation Army flag – red, yellow and blue – represent blood, fire and spirit.

– had been shamefully slow to take it seriously. While the country stacked up the worst stats in the world, its leaders including, notoriously, its Health Minister – Manto Tskabalala-Msimang – seemed unable to see what was manifestly obvious to most other countries around them. The Health Minister's comments about HIV being curable through garlic and beetroot was a source of great of embarrassment to South Africans working in this field.

Ricardo felt his own country was not the best advertisement for the approach he was championing. South Africa demonstrated that you don't have to be financially impoverished to get HIV; and that wealth and superior provision and access to information and articulate, powerful donor support doesn't make for a better AIDS response. South Africa is a rich country with a democratically elected government and free press where every one in five adults is HIV positive. How had this happened?

Ricardo tried to explain: 'South Africa differs in so many ways to the other countries. And the AIDS work here reflects a larger South African society mentality; one that still responds to a "developing world issue" as if the country were "developed". That means they rely on knowledge, expertise, literacy, education, technology, rather than the sophistication of African neighbourhood relationships. And South Africa is a proud country, happy to teach, but reluctant to learn. It'll accept advice and teaching from the Western world (and you can see evidence of this all around you) but it won't from those it assumes have a lesser experience – like Zambia or Zimbabwe, for instance. These other countries are often referred to as "those African states" (as if we are anything other than that ourselves).'

'Where does this attitude come from?'

'There are very obvious remnants of an older, more sinister conditioning of belief and practice.'

But since apartheid had been dismantled other divisions – the same old divisions – had emerged. Apartheid hadn't really been about money; it was about race (it just so happened the racists had the money). The racial divide had been dismantled but the gulf was as extreme as it ever was; new found freedoms hadn't brought the expected democratisation of wealth. Soweto illustrated this well enough. There was the tiny elite that lived in comfortable bungalows; then there was Everybody Else. Everybody Else formed a descending strata from the relatively privileged who live in monotonous rows of government-built houses with an outside tap and toilet; to the quite lucky ones who had been provided with a block of land, a prefabricated toilet and a tap, and who were allowed to build whatever they could; then the quite fortunate who lived in shacks erected in back yards; down to the squatters who built wherever they could and had virtually no facilities at all.

Kliptown was one of these places. We went there the next day with Nursing Sister Joyce Mnisi and Ricardo to meet some of the child-headed families that the Salvation Army were supporting. We turned off the main road and onto a dirt mud track and into a collection of homes in the old, slum shanty-shack style I'd seen in Nairobi's Kibera. Kliptown smelt better than the Kibera but it was just as squalid. Refuse collection seemed equally as tardy here and bags of rubbish lay all around, with dogs chewing holes in their sides. Even the worst slums have their subtle hierarchies. If anything, Kliptown lacked the vibrancy, the sheer noise of the Nairobi slum. On Soweto's Monopoly board, Kliptown would barely qualify as one of the brown properties. (Maybe Waddingtons could manufacture a Slums of the World Monopoly board – all proceeds to regeneration. NGOs could be the water and electricity boards; the churches could be stations, you pass GO and collect your ARVs.)

Sister Joyce Mnisi showed us to the houses of some child-headed families that the Army were supporting here. The house had a sofa, a television, a tape recorder, a cupboard with cutlery and three plates and mugs and a stove cooker. There was a room next to it with one double bed. This was where the girl – fifteen – slept with her younger sister and brother. She had been 'the mother' for three years now since her own mother had died from AIDS. Responsibility and loss had aged her, stolen away any lightness of being she might have had. She was weary and close to defeat. She had been helped by some financial assistance she got from the Salvation Army but her problems were not just about money, they were about time. She had none. When I asked her what she wanted most she said she wanted to be able to go out and have fun.

It was one of the more insidious side effects of this pandemic that it tied people up indoors and isolated them still further from the people around them. In the next home, we found an old, sick man who was being looked after by his wife. He was wrapped up in several blankets and hadn't been out for days. His wife was also trapped by having to tend to him and by having to look after her mentally handicapped grandson (her daughter had died of AIDS). Apart from occasional visits and support from the Salvation Army they were on their own. And what about the community? Kliptown did not seem to have the same response from within the community as other places we'd seen.

Outside, we met a man selling lollipops from a garish, makeshift portable shop. His friend 'and assistant' engaged us in chat and once he knew who we were said 'we get together as a group with our friends and talk about AIDS every week.' Joyce seemed encouraged and told the men about the monthly training that the local Corps provided and that they were welcome to attend; but this was, as Ricardo pointed out to me later, a missed opportunity and a perfect illustration of a much wider issue.

The Salvation Army had a long history of working with the people in Kliptown, and it was all very well-meaning. It was understood to be a 'mercy ministry', a 'compassionate outreach', and a 'social service'. But in Ricardo's view it did not penetrate deeply enough. It was rooted in the service provision and information and awareness approaches as opposed to the community led responses we'd seen at work elsewhere. It was a microcosm of the larger picture in the country and a hint of something that the Salvation Army itself was wrestling with: the 'we show you and help you' approach versus the 'we help you facilitate your own response' approach. Local initiative is suppressed by well-meaning service and management of the community itself into volunteers. The people should be responding out of concern for their own lives, not as volunteers of a Salvation Army programme to help them. 'This is not about our programme…it's about their lives. The question is: is it about the programme or is about the person?'

This seemed to be a fundamental battleground within the whole field of 'doing good'. Doing good for others made us feel good about ourselves because it was a charitable response; but helping people on our terms is perhaps a misplaced paternalism that stops people helping themselves (giving a man a fish instead of teaching a man to fish). And it also – crucially – prevents us, perhaps excuses us, from entering into the messy reality of other people's lives. The challenge for 'the faith guys' was that the gospel asked them to give themselves up so that they could engage with their neighbour. It came down to this: do we choose to live life behind the gates, preserve the comforts, get better security, or do we risk losing that to engage?

Later we returned to the Carl Sithole Centre. This centre, established ten years ago and named after an officer very active in the anti-apartheid movement, offered help and support to orphans. It was the first actual orphanage we had come across on the journey. Bethany Home house abandoned children between the ages of six and eighteen. The centre provided counsellors and social workers to work to help rebuild relationships with the children's families. Many of the children here – who we would meet later – were abandoned by mothers with HIV/AIDS. In a Kithituni or a Kisekele, these children might have been looked after from within the community here, but it seemed they came from a place where the communities no longer had the traditional structures, or even the will to do this.

We went to meet some orphans who got together once a week to do drama and dance and perform. They were a group ranging in age from eight to sixteen who met once a week as a kind of Sunday school. Some of the older boys were effectively fathers to the younger children in this class. The younger orphans had older children to look up to and that is literally what they were doing here, in this little spare room where the children met. There was something more painful about these older orphans. They seemed to carry a heavier burden. At least these younger orphans had older 'brothers and sisters' to look after them. But these older boys had had to try and make sense of the world on their own. It was something of a triumph that these boys were here at all. They could so easily have been somewhere else, doing something else, but they were here, learning old Zulu dances and singing *a capella* gospel and showing the other, younger orphans how to do the same.

The boys were self-conscious about us being there, but their desire to show their skill overcame that and they did a dance, all high kicks and stamping extended legs and passion. It was a beautiful and vigorous and angry dance and it seemed to us they put all their pain, anger and hope into it. Then, encouraged by our whoops and cheers, they formed a tighter circle – four of the young men led by the oldest in the centre – and they sang a song.

Even without knowing the words it was overwhelming. What were they singing about that could sound so heartfelt, so yearning, so mournful? Was it a lament for their lost youth? Was it – like the children in the field of a thousand orphans – a cry of anguish for their dead parents? Nicola asked the leader of the young quartet what that song was about. He said: 'The words are saying that when everything else in life has let you down, God is still faithful.'

Blood For Money

'The dull compulsion of the economic' – Karl Marx

In July, we left the deep purple epicentre of the pandemic and flew from South Africa to China, where HIV/AIDS was a contained but contentious issue. Although prevalence was low and evenly spread across this vast country, an intense focus on HIV/AIDS was trained on the central province of Henan, where farmers had sold unscreened blood using unsterilised equipment. To get there we took a circuitous route by train from Hong Kong to Beijing and then back south to Henan.

As our express train to Beijing pulled out of Hong Kong and curved north-eastwards at the start of its two thousand mile journey, we pressed our faces to the window, eager to catch a first glimpse of the mighty Chinese nation and to see if things – the buildings, the cars, the general shininess of Hong Kong – would dramatically change or remain the same once we had passed out of the Territories and into the mainland proper.

  I checked my new Salvation Army watch – with its red, yellow and blue striped polyester strap (indicating blood, fire and spirit) – that I had bought for the equivalent of three pounds at the Salvation Army's Booth Lodge Guest House in Hong Kong. It was 3.00 pm. In 24 hours we would be arriving in Beijing. In between, we would pass through a part of the country where half the world's manufactured goods – including my cheap watch – were made.

For the first hour there was little differentiation in the view: it was a characterless, featureless, urban sprawl – all flat topped concrete apartment blocks, bridges over brown rivers, tangled telegraph wires – as the outlying spread of two of the world's great conurbations – Hong Kong and Guangzhou (Canton) – converged. Beyond Guangzhou it became more industrial: we saw monolithic mill-house buildings that looked like old fortresses, factories with chimneys pumping dark smoke, surrounded by single-storey huts where we guessed the workers lived. The pollution from the chimneys of the factories gave the whole vista a grey-brown hue.

It was ugly but gripping. Somewhere out there men and women were making the mechanisms for my watch and a million other goods: the bicycle that Joseph and Onesmus rode around Kithituni; Major Randive's motorbike; Nicola's jeans; the England football shirt Gabriel had bought as replacement for the one he'd given Patrick; the Game Boy Agnes was playing with. This industrial complex – the engine room of the fastest growing economy on earth – was where it was all made. This was the Workshop of the World. It took nearly four hours – about four hundred miles – to get through it (our train was a very well made, fast, train. It maintained an average speed of just under one hundred miles-per-hour for the entire journey).

Outside the window the landscape began to change to flat, green fields and then to rolling hills and then to the lakes and mountains of Dongting Hu. Dusk was descending when we went to the restaurant car. We ordered chow mein from surly, smoking, hawking waiters (we were leaving a service culture and entering one just getting used to serving things as well as making them). By the time we were back in our cabin, the landscape had changed again to paddy fields that would still be there when we woke, eight hours later.

'This train is way better that the ones in England,' Gabriel said as we made up our beds for the night.

And so it was. We slept in Pullmanesque luxury: our cushioned seats converted to beds that had reading lights, cotton sheets and feather pillows. It was superlative, but was it representative? Few of the people in the countryside through which we were passing would experience luxury like this.

One essential bit of kit we had with us that was not made in China lay at the bottom of our bag, buried in the same way that we had hidden BBC mini-discs and microphones in our underpants in Zimbabwe. If in Zimbabwe we had not been able to mention the trinity of letters that make up the British Broadcasting Company; in China the prohibition extended far deeper – into the formless realms of faith itself. In Hong Kong some missionary friends had given us a couple of Bibles to pass on to their colleagues in Beijing. It was fine to own or even buy a Bible in China (it was the best-selling book there) but to pass one on equated to proselytising and openly sharing your faith in China was against the law. The books were contraband and we were Bible-runners.

That night, as we slept our hundred-mile-an-hour sleep on cotton sheets, the train passed through the central Chinese province of Henan. In a few days time we would be travelling back down to this region where, ten years ago, there had been an extraordinary and notorious outbreak of HIV/AIDS among peasant farmers. The circumstances surrounding the origins of this epidemic were still controversial enough to make our visit there a touch–and-go affair.

Before our *rendez-vous* with the Salvation Army in the capital we went to see its sites. Beijing is building at breakneck speed, choked with the smoke of construction and by the gulp of consumption. The suped-up development here – and other cities from Guangzhou to Shanghai – seems to be at a rate faster than anything ever seen. It is breathtaking. In eight years, Beijing had gone from being a largely two storey city to what we now saw from our slow-moving taxi: a skyline strutted with scaffolding, cranes and the shells of mega hotels and malls; apartment blocks in clusters, forming mini-cities; and roads clogged with slow crawling cars; conspicuous among them top-of-the-range, German saloons – always in black.

And the spark for all this creativity? Not Marx or Lenin. The new creed in China was the one most of the world worshipped – the Market. China may have been communist in word, but it was capitalist in deed. And it was not a pretty sight. The signs of the new consumerism were all around us, bursting out haphazardly, like acne on the face of a sweet-bingeing adolescent: the homeless sleeping beneath posters for Veuve Clicquot; people selling fake Rolex Oysters outside Starbucks; massive posters for Adidas football kit featuring, among others, David Beckham whose image we saw again on the subway walls of the metro at Tiananmen Square.

Meanwhile, at the entrance to the Forbidden City, an old icon: the giant-sized image of Mao Tse-tung staring out towards Tiananmen Square, over the crowds who had come to see one of China's prized treasures.

We had talked to Gabriel and Agnes about recent Chinese history and tried to explain what communism was; how it had originated in part because a man called Marx saw the terrible conditions of the workers in Britain and suggested that capitalism did not spread the wealth fairly among the poor. (Gabriel: 'I like the sharing idea, but why the no-God bit?') We had shown them the picture of Mao from the banned book *Wild Swans* by Jung Chang. We had explained how Mao had taken the ideas of communism, not because he cared about the poor (he despised them), but because he wanted power for himself. Taking my cue from Jung Chang I explained that Mao was 'possibly the greatest Mass Murderer in history'.

So, when they saw Mao's picture given such a prominent place in the square, the children were confused.

'It's the bad man,' Agnes said.

'What's *he* doing there?' Gabriel asked.

I explained that some people in China still thought well of him. Perhaps they weren't quite ready to dismantle such a potent symbol of their past. There were even people in our own country who thought Mao's image was cool.

'Maybe people don't know what he really did?' Gabriel said. He was getting the hang of how tyranny worked. Zimbabwe had been a good primer in how dictators manipulate disinformation and collective denial in order to stay in power.

'But if he killed all those people they must know something,' he reasoned.

Who knows? Perhaps the simple truth was that the people knew what he'd done but didn't want to go there. Or maybe they simply didn't have the time. China was moving so fast towards its new future there was no stopping to assess the past.

Nicola wondered if his image would still be there come the Olympics in 2008. 'That will be a true gauge of how far things have come.'

It'll be interesting to see if the world will say anything about it if he is still adorning monuments in 2008. For now, we devised our own, puerile, almost Mao-like protest. We decided that whenever we saw his picture we would say: 'Ah look, it is the Mass Murderer.'

Mao once wrote 'the country must first of all be destroyed and then reformed.' He almost succeeded in achieving the former, coercing a nation once famed for its intellectual creativity into a period of collective brain-death. In pursuing his 'philosophy' Mao was directly responsible for a peacetime death toll of seventy million people. It is an astonishing thought that in his own country this man had facilitated the deaths of nearly twice as many people as AIDS had killed in the entire world. The combination of absolute power, corrupt thinking and a cruel heart was deadlier than the worst virus known to man.

The fact that the Salvation Army is allowed to operate in China shows that things have changed. Mao had such contempt for people who had faith in anything other than himself that it is a kind of miracle Christianity survived in China at all. Mao's wife – Jiang Qing – once pronounced that Christianity in China had been consigned to the museum. She has proved to be a false prophet. The faith – mainly in the form of an indigenous, underground Church – has outlived Mao's reign and despite ongoing persecution and suppression it is still growing. In the last two decades, many of the Churches that left China during the Cultural Revolution have been able to return, if in limited, compromised form.

The Salvation Army, who have had a presence in Hong Kong since 1930, did not start work in Mainland China until 1988 when, at the invitation of the Chinese government, they were allowed to assist in emergency relief operations after an earthquake struck in Gengma, Yunnan. That event opened the door to involvement in other emergency relief and then development projects in other parts of the nation. As the country opened, opportunities for meeting need among China's poor and sick began to surface. Such was the demand (or such was the need) that in 1993, the Salvation Army opened the China Development Department in Beijing.

Puisi Chan, an energetic and dedicated woman, is the Director of this Chinese Development Department that operated from a small, tidy office tucked in one of Beijing's oldest streets. Puisi had a map of China on her office wall, stuck full of colour-coded pins indicating where the work was happening. Technically, she was managing the biggest patch of Salvation Army territory on the planet.

'There are many gaps because this country is so big,' she said. And she showed us, using the map, how she tried to plug these gaps with a small team of young men and women – all

Chinese – who made epic journeys to all parts of the nation, initiating and overseeing different projects: Child Sponsorship Development in Sichuan; micro-credit and agricultural projects in Yunnan, AIDS awareness in Kunming (almost on the border with Mizoram, India); as well as poverty alleviation in Inner Mongolia, where nomads were being re-housed in 'new cities' on the great grassland plains beyond the Great Wall. (These cities are being built because there was concern that nomads were burning wood which was causing bad air pollution in Beijing and Beijing needed to look good for the Olympics).

The red pins represented the AIDS response work and there were two – in Kunming and Longchuen in the south-west of the country. These responses were in keeping with the community driven work we'd seen elsewhere, and connected, in the main, with the usual high risk groups – intravenous drug-users and commercial sex-workers. But it was a blue pin (for micro loans response) stuck in the middle of the map in Henan Province that caught my eye.

'Shouldn't that be a red pin?'

'Yes,' Puisi replied. 'But as you know we can't operate the usual response there. We have to be careful to build it slowly. Maybe soon we can put a red pin in there.'

Had we decided to go and see the AIDS work in Kunming there would have been no difficulty in arranging the visit. The Chinese government were happy to let the Army help commercial sex-workers or drug addicts affected by HIV/AIDS; these people had got the disease through their known choices and mistakes; but Henan was different. In Henan, the local authorities had had a direct hand in bringing about the outbreak of HIV/AIDS and the resultant denial, cover up and clamp down on reporting had exacerbated the problem. Although mistakes had been admitted, accepting help there still meant admitting something that – even ten years on – the authorities found hard to do. To extend a helping hand there, the Salvation Army had to be at their most canny.

HIV/AIDS will find and expose a country's particular weakness. It had done this in every culture we'd been to so far: through India's abusive sex trade, Kenya's poverty; Rwandans brutalised society; South Africa's pride and violence; Zambia's inhumane cultural practices; fear and mismanagement in Zimbabwe. In China's lack of transparency and obsession with saving face, the virus found yet more fecund soil in which to grow. If HIV/AIDS has the capacity to bring shame and silence upon an individual; imagine what happens when that shame causes denial and obfuscation in a whole government.

Around 1998 doctors in rural regions of Henan started to report a number of patients dying from a mysterious disease. The pattern to these stories was similar in detail: a husband would fall ill, then his wife and, after a few months, both would be dead, covered in sores and dark, wine-coloured blotches. At first, no one knew what it was. But then, in 1999, a doctor called Gui Xien, an infectious diseases specialist in Wuhan University, visited some of the sick villagers and recognised their symptoms as HIV/AIDS. He immediately informed the authorities that AIDS had somehow broken out of the usual high risk groups and infiltrated the general population. What was hard to fathom was how this 'foreigners' disease' had come to infect poor rice farmers who scraped by on 2,000 Yuan ($250) a year and rarely left their villages.

Following the money yielded the answer.

In the 1980s the Chinese government launched a drive to replenish dwindling bloodbank supplies and paid donors for their plasma. For the impoverished farmers, it was not just an easy way of supplementing their income, it gave them a lifestyle farming could never provide. They could afford to build bigger houses, buy more animals; even cars; some even stopped farming altogether and became professional blood donors. A number of farmers donated blood as much as two hundred times.

The tragedy was that the needles used – some in the hands

of entrepreneurial middlemen known locally as 'blood heads' – were not always sterile. All it would need for a virus to take hold was one HIV positive donor. And that is what happened. When Doctor Gui took samples from the villagers to test them for HIV, every single one was positive. Henan health officials, reluctant to expose an outbreak that originated in a government-sponsored programme, were slow to respond and even refused to allow the doctor to return to the villages. Doctor Gui had to sneak back during the long weekend holiday and for three days he went from house to house, collecting samples, counselling patients and explaining how the virus spread.

This time he sent the report to Beijing where it was treated with the seriousness it deserved. The Henan officials were ordered to act. They could not ignore the central government's orders. Gui's whistle-blowing alerted China – and the world – to what became know as China's AIDS villages.

These were the villages we were hoping to see and it required much clandestine negotiation to get us there.

'So are we allowed to go?' I asked Puisi. We were still waiting to hear – through hidden network of communication – if we had been granted entry.

'Yes, we can all go. Daniel has arranged your visit.'

Our negotiator was a young man in his late twenties who knew people in the party in Henan. With his high cheeks and thick, spiky crop Daniel was a striking man. The fact that he was ex-Chinese army and a communist only added to his intrigue. When I asked him how it compared, Daniel said he had simply gone from one army to another. Which was true in one sense. He had gone from the largest standing army in the world to the world's most far-reaching.

Restrictions on religion allied to embarrassment and denial over what had happened in Henan all combined to make a fuzzy obfuscation necessary. Many of the AIDS villages had been off limits to the press and the officials there – many whose negligence and greed had created the nightmare – would routinely detain and expel any reporters they found. For the purposes of our visit, we would have to pretend to be something we were not. I was not a writer; I was a teacher.

In countries that fear openness, not being able to be transparent about who you are is the trade-off for being able to see something of what is going on. We'd already picked up the habit in Zimbabwe where, curiously, we had actually got our visas for China. (When the staff official at the Chinese embassy in Harare noticed in my passport that my occupation said 'writer' he asked if I was a journalist. I said no, I was a novelist. Okay, he'd said, as if that were no threat to state security.)

I rehearsed our little ruse with Gabriel and Agnes on the train as we made our seven-hour journey south with Puisi and Daniel.

'If someone asks what Mum and Dad do, then you must say we are teachers. Don't say that Dad is a writer. I'm a teacher. And Mum is a teacher.'

'Mum *is* a teacher.'

'Yes. I know. But so is Daddy.'

'Why?'

'Because the people in charge wouldn't want a writer to go there in case they wrote bad things about what happened in the place we are going to.'

'So you have to lie.'

'We have to tell a little lie so we can talk about a big lie.'

'That's silly.'

Thank God for children with their innate talent for seeing through the greyness of the adult world and their ability to state things as they actually are. What we call pragmatism; they call lying. Fair enough.

To see the AIDS villages we had to be sanctioned by, and meet the approval of, the local communist party officials there. This meant a formal banquet which was going to be both a cultural courtesy and a vetting process. The party knew our colleagues and respected them for the work they were doing; but we needed to be seen to be what we were (not now a couple of English teachers, but representatives from the donor country travelling to see how the money had been spent on social projects).

From the train we drove for forty minutes along tree-lined roads until we came to a building that looked like a large, private home but turned out to be a restaurant. Inside there were several banqueting rooms and large groups of people already at lunch. There was a great noise of laughter and shouts coming from one of the rooms and a man in a business suit emerged into the corridor as we passed through. He was completely drunk. Puisi explained that these banquets usually went on for hours and people consumed large amounts of beer or rice wine – it was quite usual and expected. She added that communist party officials were respectful of the Salvation Army's non-alcohol policy; our lunch would be a teetotal affair.

It was an easy hoop to jump through but still, nevertheless, a hoop. There were fourteen of us in all, including the mayor of the town and men and women from the Party. The men were informally dressed in short-sleeved collared shirts while the women were attired in smarter trouser suits. There was a lot of hand shaking and nodding and smiling and Puisi translated for us, explaining who we were and why we were here. We then took our seats and the food was brought out. Apart from the rice, we could not make out what any of the dishes were but they were spectacular in shape and colour and eating them was only spoilt by having them identified: chicken feet, fish stomach and sheep's eyes. Gabriel and Agnes, who had begun our journey not liking rice, tucked in bravely to anything that didn't look like an unusual animal body-part.

The conversation – translated as it was – remained superficial and polite and that seemed to suit our hosts. The mayor commented that I had 'two children' as if this were unusual (which in China it was because of the one child per family law). He said he also had two children and explained, slightly guiltily, that in the countryside, Chinese couples were allowed to have two children. It was only in the cities that the one child policy was enforced.

When we ventured questions about 'the incredible changes taking place in China,' or 'the opening up of the market and greater freedoms being enjoyed by the people' the bait was not taken. Many (perhaps mainly Westerners) were asking how communism was going to survive now that the people – party members included – had been allowed to taste the addictive fruit of capitalism (these officials had themselves arrived in a black, high spec VW Passat). But such talk was deflected. Instead we were asked about London and Britain. They all said how they would like to go there.

More food came. The revolving table in the middle of the larger table was spinning and spinning like a roulette bowl.

'Everyone is rich in the UK, yes?' This question was asked in a tone that implied being rich was a virtue.

'Not everyone. We have rich and poor like you. And a lot of people in the middle,' I said. 'But you have rich people, too.' (That month China has just overtaken the UK as the fourth largest economy in the world.)

'Yes, but how did our rich in Britain compare to rich in China?'

I said I wasn't sure. But compared to China we didn't have such a big gap between the rich and the poor. Between the people in the cities and the people in the villages.

I wanted to talk about the villages, to see if they would express an opinion but suddenly, perhaps sensing my steering, the Mayor stood up. He raised his glass and looked at me. I was asked to stand – as was custom – while he made a toast. I was now very grateful for the teetotal status of the banquet for this was the opening shot in a round of toasting that went on for about twenty minutes and involved many combinations: 'a toast to Mr Brook'; 'a toast to each person around the table', 'a toast to Mrs Brook', 'a toast to the UK'. (A toast to anything but the real reason why we were here: the good work that people were doing with the poor farmers just up the road.) How I longed for the sincere, Holy Ghost toast of Big Agnes back in Kithituni. Puisi had mentioned that the officials would use the meal as an exercise in screening and this is how it felt. It was friendly enough and the meal was generous, extravagant even; but we never got beyond the feeling we were being assessed. We must have passed some kind of test because after the toasting rounds there was a signal (a nod) from the Mayor to the party official that translated into us being free to go to both villages.

We left with a profligate amount of food uneaten. When Gabriel suggested we take some with us, knowing we were going to meet people who could use it, I said we'd better not. Taking leftover food from our banquet to poor villagers would not look good and around here looking good seemed very important.

On the way to the first village, some twenty minutes drive away, we stopped off to look at a school that had had toilets and equipment donated by the Australian Salvation Army in partnership with USAID (US Agency for International Development). There was a faded plaque, hanging on the wall of the empty school building, commemorating the day it had been opened. I hope the good people from the Australian Salvation Army and USAID would be spared the disappointment of seeing what had become of their donations.

Because the school holidays had started the place was deserted and that only added to the feeling of desolation. The school was a wreck. It had been trashed; the donated desks were all askew and dishevelled and there were no books, no equipment, not even a cupboard. In fact, it was in such a terrible state that we thought we were being shown it because it was in urgent need of attention and therefore in need of more funding from the likes of us (representatives from the donor country come to see where the money had been spent and that more might be required).

But the representative from the village – I think he was a minor official acting as liaison between the party and the project – seemed quite proud as he showed us the soiled pit latrine and urinal. Perhaps this was because he was inebriated.

I asked Puisi: 'Who did this to the classroom?'

'The children,' she said. She explained that under communism people had got so used to having things provided for them by the state that they were not used to having to take responsibility for their own possessions. It would take another generation for people to learn individual responsibility.

The only decoration in the place was a calendar, hanging lopsided, depicting the face of Mao.

'Hey, it's the Mass Murderer!' we said to each other, trusting that our inebriated guide wouldn't know what we were saying. How Mr Mao would have loved this chaos and abuse. And how he would have hated the attempts being made by a handful of individuals trying to make life better here for the 'expendable poor'.

The villages were some twenty minutes away, off the main road and set among woods next to fields where rice was grown. It was humid and overcast as we walked from the cars to the first of two villages we were allowed to see; the noise of the crickets was cacophonous.

Take away the telegraph wires and electric cables and the village could have been a set for a medieval play. The houses were well-made from small red bricks and wood. Around the houses the village had a rough perimeter wall and within the walls there were linking alleyways between the houses, where there were dogs, poultry and puddles. It was almost pretty. Unlike urban China, the village seemed to have retained some kind of intrinsic character. It had survived years of tumult – including a truly brutal recent history – but seemed just as unaffected by the soaring changes going on in the country's great cities as it had been by the Cultural Revolution.

The people's faces had a timeless quality, especially the old (and there were many of them here). They had wonderfully lined and chiselled visages, like maps of history or people in Old Masters paintings. They greeted us with warmth and far less caution than the officials back at the banquet. As we walked we gathered a crowd of men and women and the obligatory slipstream (although smaller than in Africa) of smiling, laughing children.

Despite all the attention from the outside world, the villagers had been protected from visitors. Since the epidemic had been 'outed' only a few NGOs had been allowed to operate in Henan and this was not easy (even while we were there *Médecins Sans Frontières* were in the process of pulling out after disagreements with the local authorities). There were some international foundations channelling funds here, through the local government, but the Salvation Army were the only NGO working at a community level in this village. It was a relief to get out of the bureaucratic straightjacket and stretch our legs but our walkabout still felt a bit 'monitored'.

In fairness to the authorities, they had – eventually – been very thorough in getting a supporting health system in place. In August 2005, all 280,000 farmers who had sold blood in the early 1990s were mandatorily tested by the health authorities, along with other high-risk groups. The cumulative number of HIV carriers came to 29,500 – 16,000 of which were suffering from AIDS. (The UN estimates that at the end of 2005 there were 55,000 commercial blood and plasma donors infected with HIV.)

Henan closed all unlicensed bloodbanks and all clinical supplies of blood had been screened since 1999. All the infected villagers here received free ARVs and additional medicines to treat other diseases caused by the virus. In this sense – operationally – the government had done well. And it showed a marked difference in capacity between China and a country like Kenya in being able to reach its poorest citizens. But getting ARVs to these people was not the problem. The challenge in a village like this was offering psycho-social support; giving people a hope and will to live – things provincial health programmes couldn't deliver. An effective AIDS response, though, had to treat the whole person, not just their medical and financial needs. Other needs had to be met – the emotional and (challenging here) the spiritual needs of people whose loved ones, health and livelihoods had been lost and who faced an uncertain future.

The first sign of recent, tragic events were the incongruously grand, incomplete, houses that had been built in the woodland just at the edge of the village wall. These houses had been built by farmers who – flush and sanguine with new blood money – had embarked on a building spree that got as far as the newly acquired virus within them allowed. Some of the houses had been completed, but now stood like outsized shells; their owners were either dead or no longer had the health or means to finish the work. Children – dodging, dancing, ragged children – were now using these sad mausoleums as an adventure playground.

We went to meet a family whose daughter the Salvation Army were sponsoring through school. The girl's father had discovered his positive HIV status in 2000. He looked rundown and although he was receiving the free ARVs from the government, he was not well enough to farm or do any manual work (there was no other kind available here). His condition left the family struggling to make a living and schooling a teenage daughter was beyond their means. The Salvation Army were not able to deal directly with HIV/AIDS in the manner that they did in other places – the system in Henan was not ready for a response that relied heavily on faith and community action – so they used their social-action muscles to get through and make the connections. Through child sponsorship programmes and micro-financing projects they were able to support indirectly those affected by the virus without being seen to be undermining the provincial government's own AIDS response.

The family expressed gratitude towards us all. We were symbolic visitors from the donor country and the money sent had made a difference to them. The mother was tearful as she showed us her daughter's schoolwork and she put her hands together and uttered words. Puisi said that she was 'thanking God' for the help they had received; it had given them hope. Such faith was not unusual in these parts. The walls of the family's house here were decorated with a series of red crosses against a blue background. Not Salvation Army imagery, but clearly Christian.*

On the way to the next village we passed a bar where men were playing *mahjongg* and pool. Suddenly a man started shouting at us. I put his outburst down to drunkenness (it seemed to be endemic here) but Puisi explained: 'He is saying "What about me? You didn't bring me any money last time!"' The man had to be restrained by some of the men playing pool; he did not necessarily speak for them, but his words highlighted a problem that the Salvation Army faced here: the fact that they could not give assistance to everyone in the village. Only being able to help individual cases caused some resentment. A community-based response would have got around this, but the authorities were

---

* Henan was said to be the epicentre of the underground Church that had formed during the reign of Mao and by necessity become a secret, house Church movement. A conservative estimate puts the number of Christians in China at 90 million.

not ready to permit such a thing yet; not because these people didn't have it in them (on the contrary, because of the difficulties here, the community response was more likely to succeed, when outside resources cannot be delivered so easily); but a faith-based response was out of the question. The authorities needed to be seen to be taking the lead.

Henan challenged the Salvation Army's criterion of 'integrated mission to the whole person' – it was hard in a place where the open sharing of faith was outlawed. William Booth once described the Salvation Army as being like a bird. With one wing it preached the gospel, with the other it met human needs. Unless both wings were operating, the bird wouldn't fly. China's policy of non-proselytising seriously tested this bird's capacity to get off the ground; but the Salvation Army was good at preaching without using words (as Francis of Assisi preferred it) or in Booth's language 'preaching with its hands and feet'. It was almost in the DNA of a Salvationist that to meet someone's need you sometimes had to be practical; 'You can't preach the gospel to a man dying of starvation' – or HIV/AIDS – without feeding him.

In the next village we met a man – maybe 45 years old – who lived in a one-room house, next to a pigsty. He ushered us into his room. The walls were papered with the same kitsch red crosses against a blue sky that we'd seen in the previous house. The man, whose name was Chang Su, explained how giving blood had made it possible to build a new home for his family (the unfinished shell of the house was just next door); but it had given them all a false hope. When he became sick and the money dried up, they could not finish the house and his wife left him. Then his son, embarrassed and ashamed at his father's decline, left and went to find work in the city. Although he received free medicine for his condition, Chang Su fell into despair. He was alone, had no work and felt he had nothing to live for. He was thinking of taking his own life when he received a visit from a friend who had heard that the Salvation Army were giving micro-loans to people affected by HIV/AIDS. His friend encouraged Chang Su to apply for a loan. The loan was approved and with the money he bought two pigs – now multiplied to eight. Chang Su showed us the bank draft – kept among some precious possessions – with which he had been able to buy his swine. Then he took us to see the pigs.

I never thought a pigsty could provide such a picture of hope. The sow lay suckling her six piglets in the straw and the mud and Chang Su smiled at the scene. He told us that the day he got the pigs was one of the happiest of his life. He continued to believe that God had sent his friend at the very moment he thought he might give up everything. His life had turned on this. Best of all, since getting his life back he had been reunited with his son. He pointed across the yard to where a young man of about seventeen, stripped to the waist, stood washing down the yard.

'My son came back to see me. He had heard that I had got some pigs and didn't believe it. When he saw that I was making my life again he chose to stay. Now he is working with me and we are going to get more pigs.'

It was a happy inversion of the Prodigal Son: instead of the son finding himself living like a pig and deciding to return to his father's house; here was a father seeing his son come home because the pigs had helped him live.

Out in the street two clean-cut men approached us and handed us leaflets. It was only when we reached the perimeter of the village that we saw that the leaflets were inviting people to attend a church meeting. The underground Church was not a myth. Here, right under the noses of the authorities, young men were inviting people to attend a bible meeting.

After the villages, we were treated, at the behest of the local authorities, to an accompanied tour of Henan's ancient monuments including the stunning Shao Lin Temple – the home of Kung Fu. We were put up in great comfort and some style at the Hotel Imperial in Guangzhou – a city with a fifty-storey luxury hotel completely themed around the Soccer World Cup; we were driven at high speed (in a black Audi) along impressive, newly-built motorways. Our guide and chaperone – a young woman from the local party and friend of Daniel – was kind and helpful. But none of this compared to the memory of the villages.

A few days later, we were back in Beijing and reunited with the team for a farewell lunch. Daniel and Puisi asked us about our time in the heartland of their country's ancient civilisation. We expressed out admiration and thanked Daniel for his kindness in setting up the tour, but it was the people in the village – rather than the brick-breaking monks and golden Buddhas – that we wanted to discuss. (Give us people over statues; homes over palaces.) We asked them how they felt the visit had gone. I had watched Daniel during the walkabout and noticed how connected and how moved he was by the experience. He had a number of qualities – he was calm, he was patient, he was organised – but compassion was what he had in abundance. Puisi had mentioned how much Daniel had changed since starting to work for the department. 'I invited him to help the project as local staff to work in this project from a hospital support group network. He first started as part-time and later moved to full-time project staff for Henan project. His behaviour and attitude started changing dramatically after he participated in our work. The work changes you.'

So how had this ex-Chinese Army and communist party member come to work for the Salvation Army, a Christian army? I asked Puisi to ask Daniel.

'He says he liked what he saw. The work. He liked seeing how we were helping people.'

'But he could do this – with other organisations, with an NGO. Why do it with you? What is his motivation?'

Puisi asked him the question and Daniel laughed. Then he blushed and gave us his answer, in English:

'Am I allowed to say "God"?'

Servants and Stars

'I wasn't a drug addict, I was a slut'
– Gill (a resident at Allegria house)

On the last leg of our journey, we travelled to Los Angeles and the part of the world with which the acronym HIV/AIDS first became associated: the west coast cities of the United States.

We drove east along Sunset Boulevard, Los Angeles – a road, a strip, pregnant with glamour and carnality – to do our final piece of official work: a visit to a Salvation Army HIV/AIDS housing project called Allegria House. It was an unexpected but fitting road upon which to end our epic journey. We were pointing homewards (if we just kept going we'd get there eventually) and the pull of home and friends and family was powerful now. And the USA – in our memories at least – was the country where HIV/AIDS had first appeared, among the gay communities of San Francisco, New York and here in Los Angeles over twenty years ago.

Allegria lay at the tatty end of the Boulevard where it petered out into the homogeneity of junk-food and commercial premises, through the new immigrant populations of Chinese and then the Spanish neighbourhoods. On the way we passed through the different strata of American society, from privilege to impoverishment in a 25 mile stretch. Sunset is working-girl turf, tourist trap, immigrant haven and home to some of the world's most glamorous people.

At the western end of the road, in Beverly Hills, putting-green-flat lawns front ostentatious but secluded houses – the homes of the stars. Somewhere up there, among the palms and bougainvillea, was 'The Castle' – the former home of the actor Rock Hudson – the first person I can remember dying of a disease called AIDS; maybe the first person to give the disease 'a face'. I can clearly recall that face – the gaunt, sunken features of the man who had once been the 'epitome of handsome' – appearing on the news.

Back in 1984, there was still a Chinese-like reticence and whisper surrounding the disease – a lack of clarity that lasted for several years. Even when Hudson was diagnosed as being HIV positive, his publicity staff and doctors – perhaps fearing he would become ostracised in the Hollywood community if they had known the truth about his condition and his sexuality – told the public he had liver cancer. A month later, he issued a press release saying that he was dying of Acquired Immunodeficiency Syndrome – and that he was homosexual. But in a later press release, Hudson speculated he might have contracted HIV through transfused blood from an infected donor during the multiple blood transfusions he received as part of his heart bypass procedure. Only after his death – in a spat of recrimination between his ex-lovers – was the connection made between Hudson's sexual activity and the acquiring of the disease.

Shortly before his death, Hudson stated, 'I am not happy that I have AIDS. But if that is helping others, I can at least know that my own misfortune has had some positive worth.' Rather than pull down some of the veils surrounding AIDS, it seems Hudson's 'partial confession' had a reverse affect, restricted as it was by fear of two different prejudices: one against homosexuality, the other against a disease that people didn't understand. For a time the double stigma of being homosexual and having AIDS became synonymous and this lured the world into thinking HIV was a 'gay disease' (I remember the jokes at the time constructing crude alternative acronyms for AIDS – Question: What does AIDS stand for? Answer: Anal Injected Death Syndrome). AIDS, as far as the Western world was concerned – became the gay disease and the deaths of other high-profile gay men – the musician Freddie Mercury, the writer Bruce Chatwin* – seemed to reinforce this idea. Some say that it wasn't until the basketball star Magic Johnson – a black, heterosexual athlete – admitted he was HIV at a press conference in 1991, that perceptions of AIDS in the American people's thinking changed. In a nation that looked to its stars for guidance, it took one of its biggest to kill off the 'gay disease' tag.

In those early years, serving people with AIDS was retarded by the sexuality issue as much as it was by ignorance about the actual virus; people did not want to touch someone with AIDS for fear of infection. While some were quick to condemn, those on a firmer ground did something to help. The Salvation Army at that time were already working among the sex-workers and drug-users (many of them gay) in the cities where AIDS appeared and, as a natural consequence of their work, found themselves doing what they always did – ministering to the whole needs of a person without prejudice. Dr Ian Campbell (who at this time was working in the hospital in Chikankata, Zambia, where men and women were presenting with AIDS-like symptoms) was watching development in America closely for clues as to how to respond.

---

* The travel-writer, Bruce Chatwin, once wrote a story (collected in *What Am I Doing Here?*) called 'Until My Blood Is Pure' about a man who had contracted a sexually transmitted disease and waits in an African country to see a doctor in the vain hope that he might clear himself of the infection before returning home to his wife. Chatwin died of 'pneumonia' in 1989. He said he had succumbed to a rare exotic illness, 'a fungus' he picked up from inhaling dust on a trip to China; or perhaps a bird flu from Hong Kong. Despite his dissembling, others knew he had AIDS. He did once declare that he was going to Africa to 'find a stable form of the HIV virus and the Aga Khan was to be approached for funding.' But Chatwin never really 'went there.' A few years after his death the real cause of his death was revealed to be HIV/AIDS.

Apart from noting the epidemiological similarities, what he saw in the gay community's response to the epidemic gave him hope: 'I noted the strength of the gay response to HIV and AIDS in San Francisco when I was in Zambia. If they – an isolated and, at that time, ostracised group of people – could help each other then think how a close community with multigenerational families close at hand might respond. It gave us hope for a communal response so we went for it.'

Without looking for it, the Salvation Army had found itself at the front line of an epidemic that would very soon become a pandemic. They were the first organisation to extend a helping hand to those communities at a time when the shunning of the infected was at its peak and because they were already on the ground, working with drug-users and sex-workers, they were among the first to see the disease cross over from the perceived high risk groups and into the family.

Allegria House was a housing project, purpose-built yet beautifully designed to accommodate families whose members were HIV positive (sometimes it might be the mother, sometimes the child, sometimes the whole family.) The director of the project, Jeffery Lane, showed us around the accommodation and it felt like a tour he was only too happy to conduct. Allegria was a well-conceived and mindful construction: a place someone would want to live. The whole ambience, from the bright colours of the houses to the sound of children playing in the yard, conveyed this. Allegria means happiness or joy in Spanish. Jeffery explained: 'We try to capture that. Even though people have this disease, we want them to make the best of their life.'

Allegria served about 180 people a day on the campus. Most people here stayed an average of nine months, although the families in permanent shelter (a modest description) could stay as long as they felt necessary. Jeffery explained that many people came in from the street with nothing so everything was supplied:

from clothes to furniture. Maybe, such a project could have only been realised in donor-rich America but the spirit of it – giving the very best standard of accommodation and facilities to the poorest – reminded me of Dr Paul Farmer's approach to medical treatment in Third World countries: the preferential treatment of the poor, whatever it costs. The extravagance of it said more clearly than words what was valued here.

'Surely no one would ever want to leave?'

'No. But they get to a place where they want to leave – where they can. They get to a place where they are restored enough to want to move on.'

Gill was a mother of two in her thirties, who had been living in Allegria for three months by the time we met her. She ushered us into her apartment – which was immaculate and lived-in – and sat us down to hear her story. She was, she explained, 'a woman turned around'. Her story was harrowing but she told it in such a frank, self-disclosing way that it was impossible to feel sorry for her or detect any self-pity.

'I had some emotional problems relating to my AIDS status. Let's put it this way: I was blown out of the water when I discovered my status in July 2004. I was four months pregnant. When my daughter was born, she was diagnosed HIV as well. When she was treated at UCLA, they referred me to Allegria. I don't know where I'd be without them.'

'You know how you got it?'

'Yeah. After the shock, I knew how I'd got it. That was obvious. People presumed I was a drug-user. A lot of people still didn't think you could get this from heterosexual sex. They'd see me and then ask me "How long have you been clean?" I'd say "Hey I've been clean all my life. I was never a drug addict… I was a slut!"'

I don't think I'd heard anyone on the journey state how they got the virus as boldly as this. It was clear to see and hear the connection between Gill's lack of self-pity and her recognising that she'd acquired HIV through her own actions. It wasn't just a brash personality; this ability to be bold – transparent – came out of the acceptance she'd found at Allegria.

'When I discovered my status I wanted to talk about it but I had to be careful. People would say "Hey, you mean you got it like Magic Johnson." They'd say that poem: "Take the 'I' out of HIV and 'I' is still me." I'd just say, "Hey, you don't even have to screw around as much as Magic did to get HIV!"

I'm still careful about who I talk to. Some get it; some don't. Some still cross-up like you're a leper. Someone last year asked me if they could contract it through sharing a glass with me! We still have some way to go. Also I didn't want to blab about it because of my children. I didn't want to put my crap on my fifteen-year-old daughter. But in Allegria you don't have to keep quiet. You don't have to keep it a big secret. It's pretty helpful being able to say to your neighbour, "Hey, you try this or that medication?" Sure, some people keep it to themselves. Some parents here don't disclose but eventually most people get to a place of being comfortable enough to declare their status. I can't tell you what a thing that is. Like dumping a heavy bag.'

Gill showed me a picture of her daughter. 'Here she is. You know, I look back on my life and all the things that were important to me then and now they are irrelevant. Now it's the little things, day-to-day things, that make all the difference. People used to say that to me and I never believed it. I believe it now.'

As we walked through the gardens to meet the Project Director, I asked Jeffery where he thought AIDS was at in the USA and what his thinking on it was.

'You get two responses: people are tired of it. They fatigue of hearing about it. Isn't that over with now? Then there's the fact that people are still unsure of how the disease affects people and society. It's really the first post-modern plague and it has a lot of things – difficult things – to teach us. It can give us insights about what this next part of earth's history is going to be. There's this paradox at the heart of it. Nothing is more personal than how HIV is contracted; but it's a global disease. So we have to ask, how do we respond to this? Especially when people have turned off things that are power oriented – churches, politicians – you have to find new ways of reaching them. The key is getting to the root of what people are searching for in the first place. Sex and drugs are part of that search and they can only fill the void for so long. What do they really need to fill the void with? We have to get to the root of these questions because otherwise all we're doing here is managing a disease – keeping sick people alive, instead of dealing with the issue of true health and healing – which includes the body but goes beyond it.'

We finished the tour by talking with Julie, the Programme Director at Allegria.

I asked her what the key ingredient in this programme was.

'You should embrace people with love, a measure of grace, kindness and compassion. This disease makes people feel unworthy and lonely. They get isolated. And this affects their health. Whether they live in Park Avenue or on a park bench, their health is affected by the way they feel about themselves. Sometimes we forget this because we can give people drugs. Whether you're in the richest or poorest country, the principle is the same. People need to feel life is worth living. It would be good to find a cure for this thing but it wouldn't solve the issue of how people get there in the first place and it shouldn't change how we respond to people who have it.

I'd like to see the love we have to give as being contagious. Love is the best antidote we currently have.'

Someone – a film producer, I think – once said if it's a good story you should be able to get it down to one sentence. In the last weeks of the journey we had begun to try and compress our experience into a tight little summarised ball – not so much to pitch a film but so as to have a ready answer to bounce back at the question I knew we were going to be asked by friends and family upon our return: 'How was it?' Time would be short, people's attention spans would be limited. So, maybe it was a good idea to have a short, ready answer to hand.

As we passed by the MGM Studios on our way to LAX Airport, I imagined trying out my summary on the studio executives there. I pictured myself walking into a light, clean office dressed in my dirty, split shorts and khaki T-shirt and, for added effect, the walking shoes I had worn pretty much every day for the last nine months and that still had the red dust of Africa in the grips. Across the table I faced fresh-laundered, strong-cologned executives looking for stories to tell and sell.

'So. What's the big story?'

'Well, the big story is really lots of little stories.'

'How does it start?'

'It starts with a white, middle-class family leaving their comfortable home and going to places affected by HIV/AIDS and…'

'Something really bad happens to one of them?'

'It's not really about us. There are lots of characters.'

'Yeah, but who's the hero?'

'There are lots of heroes.'

'But who's the star?'

'No stars. Just servants.'

'Servants? People don't want to see servants. Where's this thing set? We need locations nailed down.'

'Well, it starts in Africa, moves to India…but it's really not a fixed geography.'

'Africa? Too depressing. Unless it's a conspiracy. Or a safari. But no one here wants to see that African suffering shit. Anywhere else. You say you went to India?'

'I have stories from India. There was a man there looking after the children of the sex-workers in a rough town and he almost single-handedly…'

'Prostitutes and children! It's not going to play in Boise, Idaho.'

'Does he have to be Indian? Any Americans?'

'Well, yes. There were a few. In particular there was this one American woman who worked in the AIDS response work for the Salvation Army, in Kenya.'

'The Salvation Army? Does it have to be about them? They suck. All those charity stores? Come on. Let's make something sexier than that. Even the UN is sexier than that.'

'Well…'

'And did you say AIDS? We're all done with that. *Philadelphia*. Tom Hanks. We covered that. We don't want more movies about suffering.'

'It's not about suffering. It's about…'

'And AIDS – half the actors here aren't available because they're doing some AIDS charity work somewhere – Angelina, Brad – they're all at it. They should stick to what they do best. It's getting too much. Anyway. I still don't hear the story, Mr Brook. Narrow it down. Be specific. Summarise the journey for me, in a sentence. Everyone knows if it's great it can be told in a sentence. That's what McKee says.'

'Ok. The world is in very bad shape but it's being held together by small acts of kindness.'

Silence.

'Is that it?'

'In a sentence.'

'I don't know if that's enough of a story. Where's the bang, the conflict, the arc? Where's the jeopardy? People are looking to escape. They want to leave the theatre feeling good not wanting to kill themselves. They need to be uplifted. They need good news!'

'That is the good news.'

'I don't see it. I'm sorry. I just don't see it.'

And the Way Out?

'You already know enough. So do I. It is not knowledge we lack. What is missing is the courage to understand what we know and to draw conclusions.'
– Sven Lindqvist

The first day we got home, Gabriel and I walked up the Upper Richmond Road to see if it was still there; and to see what it felt like to simply walk to a shop, buy a coffee, get some money from a cash machine, buy a paper and spend a day not thinking about or being confronted with the poor state of the world.

'I wonder if we'll meet someone we know,' Gabriel said.

That prospect had me slightly agitated. I wasn't sure if I was ready for the inevitable, 'So-how-was-the-trip?'; not sure if I was prepared to compress nine months of life-changing experience into one glib sentence for someone who was on their way to buy some Kenyan *mange-tout* from Waitrose. But it was the end of August and the schools were on holiday and the usually car-crammed street was quiet; maybe we'd be able to sneak there and back without having to give an account of ourselves.

As we passed East Sheen Primary, Gabriel craned his neck to see if his school had changed in any way. 'Looks the same.' His tone was exactly half way between pleased and disappointed. We passed the corner shop, the antique shop, the café, and the garden centre – all still there; also pleasingly and disappointingly unchanged.

While we had been away having our most basic assumptions challenged, it seemed life in this little patch of West London had continued unruffled. People still purchased lottery tickets and lemon trees; there were three new loft conversions under way. It was, as the author of *The Innocent Anthropologist* – Nigel Barley – said of coming back home after living in a mud hut for a year: 'positively insulting how well the world functions without one.'

By the time we reached Blockbuster Video Gabriel said: 'Dad, it feels like we haven't been away. Like we didn't see all those things. It's weird. I can't describe it.'

I reassured him: 'I know what you mean. It's okay. It's normal to feel that.'

Gabriel was having the bittersweet, existential moment all returning travellers have when they confront the normality of home. Bitter because home, by its very familiarity and sameness, mocks the adventurer with: 'So you travelled the world; you saw some stuff. We managed perfectly well without you.' And sweet because this predictable, peaceful, protected normality was precisely what we wanted home to be to us. Normality was what we longed for when we were scrabbling by torchlight to a pit-latrine in the middle of the night; or throwing up into an Indian Airways sick-bag; or when we no longer had the energy to explain ourselves to a gathered village; normality was not having to think about AIDS or poverty or the troubles of the world every day.

We were almost at the cash point – home free – when we were ambushed by, of all things, an advertising hoarding. Right there, on the side of Blockbuster Video's wall, stood a massive billboard featuring a beautiful, smiling supermodel and a beautiful, laughing Masai warrior.

'Masai,' Gabriel said.

('Good,' I thought. 'That was something he didn't know before the trip.')

It was an advertisement for American Express RED – the campaign I had actually read about sitting in Other Agnes' café in Kithituni at the beginning of the year. RED was the initiative – launched by rock star Bono and businessman Bobby Shriver – designed to help fight AIDS in Africa. For every pound spent on the card, American Express contributed a minimum of 1% to the Global Fund.

The poster got me all stirred up. Just when I thought we were going to have a conscience-free stroll to latte-land, this big advert goes and spoils my day. In my head I spewed all my best, newly informed 'seen-it-done-it-I-know-what-I'm-talking-about-now' put-downs: Is that the best we can do? Fight AIDS with shopping? Is that the solution we have for everything now? The commoditisation of a virus? Has it just become another industry? And what's with the happy smile and the healthy skin and teeth? The last Masai warrior we had seen had been driving his skinny, half-dead cattle alongside the Mombasa Highway in search of grass. And why do we need celebrities to tell us what to do? And since when was it about money? And this isn't engagement this is…'

In my pompous indignation, I almost failed to see the poster for what it was: a fairly brave if uncomfortable attempt to build a bridge between consumerism and conscience.

Gabriel read the headline: '"My card; my life," What's it for?'

'Oh, I don't know…it's…encouraging people to use a credit card so when they buy things some of the money goes to help people with AIDS.'

Detecting my tone Gabriel asked 'What's wrong with that?'

'Nothing.'

Nothing. For most people, giving money was as close to engagement as they were going to get. And this campaign was a step on from being 'charity'. The companies involved would make profit and that made their involvement sustainable. The people who'd had the idea for the campaign had already worked out that to get things done you have to work with what you've got. Use one tidal wave to counter another. You can't ask people to stop shopping, so meet them where they are and catch the crumbs from their shopping baskets.

Meet people where they are. Don't tell them what to do. Do the thing that you can. Work with what you've got. Hadn't our whole journey taught us the importance of these things? Come on, Brook. Why not try and apply the lesson in your own life?

'So how was the trip?'

Our friends – Lucy and Andy – had got us round for dinner specifically to hear all about it. There was time to give more than my pithy, McKee-proof sentence, honed to fit the expediency of modern living – 'The world is in terrible shape and its being held together by small acts of kindness' – and which I had tried out a few times with a neighbour in our street and with the staff in Oddbins Wine Merchants where I had bought the chilled bottle of Chablis we were now drinking (silently thanking God for refrigeration, electricity, a liveable wage and wine growers). While they poured out the wine they let us pour out our recollections and opinions; they even let us show our photographs. Then, after dinner, having listened to the unedited, tumbling tale of our travels, Andy's father Chris Mayfield – the former bishop of Manchester – asked an exacting question:

'So what?'

The question hung in the air. Wow. Back only three days and the heroic and humble adventurers have to face a question like that. Can't we have a few more weeks of praise and awed looks of admiration?

'Well. We need to tell people about what we saw. And I have to write about it. Bear witness.'

'Good. And then?'

And then. And then. The ex-Bishop hadn't asked the question in a belittling or dismissive way; it was the sincere prompt of a man used to asking himself 'How do I turn words into deeds?'; exegesis into praxis? I knew where he was taking me. What are you going to do – after the words, the talks, the slideshows, the radio broadcasts, the book and – who knows? – the film? – with what you have seen?

Telling people about the problem is the easy part. The trick is being able to do something about it.

It is easy to describe the problem and then sit back thinking you've done your bit while your imagined audience, moved by your words, changes the world. 'Bearing witness' – the writerly duty of providing the pure unsullied evidence through words – is such a noble-sounding calling; it has a kind of impregnable moral authority about it; what more can you do than present and describe what you've seen? In fact, for writers, doing more than bearing witness is regarded as being in bad taste – and worst – bad writing. Writers should describe what they see (and to muse at what they can't) but if they happen to have insight in to what might be 'an answer' to a problem in the world then it is best to disguise it as a question and let the almost-answer hang enigmatically, tantalisingly just out of reach. (The use of 'maybe' and 'perhaps' – two words I fear I've used a lot in this book – indicate this technique.) A writer can suggest, but one thing he must never do is tell people what to do. Only madmen, prophets and busybodies do that.

William Booth – a man accused of being all three – had no pretensions to be a writer (*In Darkest England* was co-written with journalist W. T. Stead) although some of its passages wouldn't look out of place in *Hard Times* (Dickens wasn't afraid of being didactic) and Tolstoy copied the ideas (and title) for his own book of plans for social reform (*In Darkest Russia and the Way Out*). Free of this particular vanity, Booth was able to break the good 'writing' rule and not only describe the sickness but dare to offer diagnoses, maybe even cure. Having described – in authoritative detail – the scale of the poverty, alcoholism and prostitution faced by the 'submerged tenth' in London

and England in the first part of the book; in the second part –
...*and the Way Out* – he proposed a number of practical solutions
that seem so prescient now (citizens advice, affordable housing,
free medical care for the poor) it's amazing to think he was
ridiculed for suggesting such things. I often wondered what
scheme Booth would have come up with if AIDS and not alcohol
was the prime killer of his time.

If the scoffers objected to Booth's ideas it was probably less to
do with the quality of the social reform he suggested than the
fact that Booth had a spiritual motivation and perspective. As a
Christian, Booth believed that the world was in a fallen state,
needed redemption; had already been redeemed by a Redeemer;
and was in a process of being redeemed by people who believed
in that Redeemer. It was perfectly natural for him to believe that
there was a spiritual solution to physical problems because for
him the body and the soul; the material and the spiritual were not
separate. A Christian should take the soul as seriously as the body
and the body as seriously as the soul. Somewhere in our history
– Plato gets the blame – a dualism (a separation of body and soul)
occurred and it has informed the way we see the world ever since.
This has consequences for how we see health and sickness, life
and death. And it has relevance for the way we respond to AIDS
(and pretty much any form of suffering).

Before setting off on this journey all the noise around this
disease seemed to be about money, condoms and drugs and
how to distribute them. While few out in the field would argue
that these things are not important, the acquiring and spread of
AIDS can't just be attributed to a lack of the above; just as our
response to AIDS can't just be a logistical question of how we
disseminate 'stuff'. As we saw, AIDS isn't just a medical problem,
it is an environmental problem (clean water, need for power); an
economic and social problem (education, roads, infrastructure,
medical care); and it is a spiritual problem (it is formed through
relationships and its antidote is found through relationships).

What programme can give hope to a community struggling with grief and loss; or make a man who is dying feel his life worth living? How do you help people asking the question what it means to really be alive? Or what happens when I die? What scheme or programme can make a person feel loved, supported, wanted, dignified?

What gives someone with nothing the ability to save a tiny amount of money a month in order to purchase something that will help them and others; where does a person get the motivation to walk ten miles to see someone who is sick without being paid to do it?

These are spiritual questions.

The supplying of drugs, money, information and condoms may constitute the visible signs of a response to the pandemic but it is the hope that comes from faith – as a dynamic experience (not a dead doctrine) that constantly made the difference wherever we went. Not faith in the donor, the politician or the celebrity, but faith in an unseen, invisible God who some believe really enters into the sickness, the slum, the infected, the rejected. So many of the small stories were part of this big story and the proof of it was this vast, usually unsung, often unseen, unplanned network of small acts of kindness – the glue that bound it all together.

After a few weeks, we were back into the rhythms of the old life; swallowed whole by work and school, the multiple, sophisticated concerns that make our privileged and blessed lives here so complicated. We were back to grabbing what snatched time our business allowed us, our conversations became more truncated, our African graces of gratitude for water, gas, cars, DVDs and health got shorter; the trip became a fading memory.

In an effort to subvert this trend we did a series of slide shows at our house for people from our community. We had taken a lot of pictures on the journey half knowing that, at some point in the future, some of these photographs might appear in a book or perhaps a slide show. As I took these pictures, I had told myself that they should be more than the glorified holiday snaps of a well-travelled family, but a part of the 'bearing witness' – a way of helping people understand; more than a record of doom; but a gallery of hope. It was time to test this out.

As the pictures were beamed up onto the living room wall, I watched the faces of the watching people, hoping that we were not merely adding to the pornography of catastrophe people already got from the news; hoping that they'd see beyond the poverty, the disease, the suffering, to the things in-between. Here's the bad news but can you see the good? I feared the distressing pictures would be more interesting than the hopeful ones; that the shot of the people lying on a sheet in the street, or the disgusting fascination of a city without toilets would linger longer than the smiling faces of the old widow or the young orphan; but it wasn't the case. The people in the room responded to the people on the wall and, in a long range act of communion, I called out their names as their faces appeared:' Big Agnes, Jonathan, Mark, April, Onesmus, Johnnie Boy, Georgie-Porgie, Joseph, Anton, Jacob, Margaret, Martin, Abednego, Oral Robert, Mama Safi, Other Agnes, Major Randive, Ratnamala, Priyanka, George, Jimmy, Meble, Beatrice, Celestine, Augustus, Joseph M, Jackson, Pascal, Martha, Ricardo, Puisi…' Each one a story deserving of more than this; but each one part of the chain – the glue – that made up the big story.

After the pictures the people asked questions.

What had we learned?

The world is in terrible shape, but we always knew that. Money isn't the answer, but we always suspected that. Mankind gets its priorities badly wrong, but that's not a surprise.

Gratitude.

And that it's not about doing good for others, but learning how to be good with others.

Was it hard settling back? It was easier than we thought –

especially for the children who have this ability to live in the present. But ask us in a year.

What do you miss? We miss the simplicity but not the poverty. We miss the walking but not the bad roads; the children laughing but not the lack of schools. We miss the praying but not the three-hour church services. We miss the sunshine but not the drought.

What can we do?

There are organisations you can support. You might even go and see it for yourself.

Does faith really make a difference?

Yes.

Had we changed?

I think so, but change is hard to see. Ask us in a year.

What would you say is the most important thing?

It is about being 'present' wherever you are.

As people asked the questions I began to realise that they weren't just asking them in the context of what they might do to help 'those people'; they were asking, 'What can we do to help each other?' After a while, people started to answer each other's questions across the room and for a time our house became a rondaval and the middle-class people of South West London a tribe voicing their own anxieties and fears: are we living in the right way? Should we do more? Should we challenge our own cultural practises? Can we change? What do we put our hope in? They were questions people really wanted answers to – the questions the people in the room were thinking about: our deep fears and concerns, anxieties about aspirations and hopes, about what we long for, what we do with our lives, what happens when we die? The questions we almost don't allow ourselves to ask because we don't have the time or because there is little forum for doing such things.

At the end of the evening, someone put up their hand and said: 'Hey, isn't this a community conversation?'

Just before leaving Kithituni Jonathan Mutungwa had said to me 'Tell your people about us.' He was giving us permission to tell their story, show the pictures, talk about them, write about them. This instruction might have been motivated by the simple human desire to be known and not be forgotten (like Pascal's request to write his name somewhere). But Jonathan didn't say it like that. It wasn't 'Tell your people how bad things are here and get them to send money;' it was quite the reverse. His inflexion was that of a man saying – 'Tell them the good news about us; spread the rumour.' He had never been to London, nor even seen what life was like outside Kenya, but he could tell that his story had something in it that mattered to communities beyond his own. 'What has happened to us here in these last few years has reminded us of what matters. Tell people about us and you will remind them of what matters.' He knew that what we had seen in his community contained a secret worth passing on, a story that wasn't just about how to deal with this pandemic or what to do about people who are dying; but a story about how to live a life.

Acknowledgments

Thanks must go to:

Nikki Capp for hoping for things unseen; Ian and Alison Campbell for being pioneers and mentors; Sue Lucas, Don Odegaard, Charles King and Pauline Stevenson-Baker for their expertise.

Andy York and my godfather, Jeff Barker, for wise counsel; Robert Butler and Simon Willis for suggesting me; James McManus for being practical; Rupert Murdoch for saying yes.

April Foster for her friendship and house; Meble for behind the scenes cover; Sherry and Paul Pelletier for back-up; Rebecca Nzuki for getting outside the city gates.

The people of Kithituni for their largesse, in particular the magnificent Mutungwa family for taking us in as their own: Mark; Jonathan and Agnes; Jacob and Margaret, Richard and Martin; Henry; Abednego, Catherine and Kevin.

For joy, pain and mangoes on the road: Onesmus, Johnnie Boy, Joseph, Georgie-Porgie, Oral Roberts, Anton and the rest of the local response team, including the beautiful widows.

Agnes (the Café); Lucas; Jackson; Lelu for keeping us in water; George (the Baptist) and family; Rhoda Kyengo; Sylvester; and Mama Safi, Majors James and Grace.

Douglas; and Commissioner Hezekial Anzeze.

Pierre Robert for unburdening me of my shorts.

Major Randive, his wife Ratnamala and daughter Priyanka; Pravin; Timothy; Sunita; Nishikant Rananaware.

Jimmy and George and the CHAN team.

For hosting and giving up their beds: Majors Joash and Florence Malabi; Captains Beatrice and Celestine; Nicodeme and Janvier. Also Alphonsene and Marie Rose; and Ainea Kimaro.

For his skill, Joseph Malakisi; for his calm Major Augustus Webaale.

The Nduati family; and Compassion.

Captain Kennedy for driving safe; and Captain Angela Hachitapika for remembering the story.

For refuge in a difficult time: Tim and Sam Johnson; Bob and Marguerite Ward; and Ian Swan.

For stylish, witty and thoughtful accompaniment, Ricardo Walters; Major Lenah Jwili and Joyce Minisi; and Nomsa.

For rest and reminder: Jackie Pullinger, Margaret, Lina Duncan and all at the St Stephens' Society.

For tireless commitment: Puisi Chan and the team, including Daniel. For air-con and World Cup TV, Amanda Ericcson and the gang. And in the USA: Jeffery Lane.

I also want to thank:

My publisher Catheryn Kilgarriff and the staff at Marion Boyars for backing me before I'd even packed and not letting me get away with anything.

Our friends at the South West London Vineyard for providing five star 'cover'.

And thanks to the incredible Blacker family for putting us up and getting us raw and making us tell their neighbours...

The BBC World Service for giving me a mini-disc and letting me use it without a microphone. Stuart Buckman for setting it up.

Christine Morgan and the rest of the 'Thought for the Day' producers for risking long-range, live broadcasts. The 'Today' programme for air-time. As well as Juliette Howell and the team at Maverick TV for wanting to make the story before knowing what it was.

And thanks to my incredible family: my amazing wife Nicola for seeing it before I did; and to my two extraordinary children – Gabriel and Agnes – who usually saw things as they actually were and said so.

And thanks to the Lord who makes something good of unpromising material; for instigating a plan and letting us be a part of it.

Bibliography

Barley, N. (1983) *The Innocent Anthropologist.* London: British Museum Publications

Booth, W. (1891) *In Darkest England and the Way Out*, London: Salvationist Publishing and Supplies

Chang, J. (1996) *Wild Swans,* London: HarperCollins

Chatwin, B. (2005) *What Am I Doing Here?*, London: Random House

Gourevitch, P. (1998) *We Wish To Inform You That Tomorrow We Will Be Killed With Our Families,* New York: Farrar, Straus & Giroux

Kidder, T. (2003) *Mountains Beyond Mountains,* London: Random House

Kipling, R. (1993) 'The Elephant's Child' *Just So Stories,* London, Wordsworth Editions

Lindqvist, S. (1997) 'Exterminate All The Brutes.' London, Granta Books

Murphy, D. (1994) *The Ukimwe Road*, London: HarperCollins.

Naipaul, V.S. (1977) *India: A Wounded Civilization*, London: Andre Deutsch

Sontag, S. (1989) *Aids and its Metaphors*, New York: Farrar, Straus & Giroux

Thomas R.S. (2000) 'The Welsh Hill Country,' *Collected Poems 1945-1990*, London: Phoenix

Wallace, J. (2000) *Faith Works*, London: Random House

If you would like to engage in the HIV/AIDS response work described in this book then please contact:

IHQ-IntHealth@salvationarmy.org

or

www.salvationarmy.org.

For child sponsorship:

Compassion at: www.compassionuk.org.